Contents

BOOK NO: 1786773

Breaking Bad News

Establishing an Auditable Procedure for Giving the Cancer Diagnosis

G Walker, J Bradburn & J Maher

*Lynda Jackson MacMillan Centre for Cancer Support and Information,
Mount Vernon Hospital, Northwood*

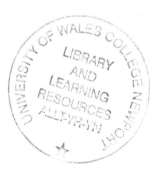

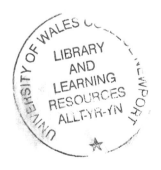

King's Fund

Published by
King's Fund Publishing
11–13 Cavendish Square
London W1M 0AN

ISBN 1 85717 135 7

A CIP catalogue record for this book is available from the British Library

Distributed by Bournemouth English Book Centre (BEBC)
PO Box 1496
Poole
Dorset
BH12 3YD
Tel: 0800 262260
Fax: 0800 262266

Printed and bound in Great Britain

*Breaking Bad News – Guidelines and Patient Information
Card* is available from Pat Tawn on 0171 307 2672.
Price £2.00

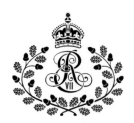

Acknowledgements

The research team would like to thank the following people:

The King's Fund for the grant which enabled the project to take place, and for their interest at all stages.

Dr Jane Maher, on whose original idea the project was based, for her enthusiasm, encouragement and powers of negotiation.

The members of Luton & Dunstable CARE; Caritas Self Help Cancer Group Harrow; Stevenage Cancer Support Group; Chiltern Breast Care Support Group.

Jane Millan, Cherry Mackie, Joan Timlett, Paul Cole, Ian Chait, Brian Shorey, Vic Robinson, Sheila Small and Judy Young, who were all members of the joint working group.

The patients and doctors who were interviewed for giving so freely of their own experiences.

All those involved in the piloting and auditing of the guidelines, especially Alvin Pope, John Ochai and Julie Joyce.

Angela Hall for her help and encouragement in the early stages of the project.

The clinical audit departments at both Mount Vernon and Watford General Hospitals.

Ann Swallow for enabling us to complete the final report and for organising the finances.

The staff of the Lynda Jackson Macmillan Centre for their support and encouragement.

Executive summary

This study aimed to involve patients and health professionals in drawing up a set of auditable guidelines for consultations in which patients are given their initial diagnosis of cancer. It resulted from representations from patients and hospital staff, both of which groups were concerned that the way in which the diagnosis was given was often less than satisfactory, and could prejudice the patient's future emotional well-being. These concerns coincided with the publication of an Audit Commission report on communication between hospitals and patients, which emphasised the importance of organisational aspects of communication.

The study was based in three hospitals and took place in three stages:

1   Data gathering
    – literature review
    – review of current practice
    – feedback from patients using interviews and focus groups
    – feedback from consultants using interviews

2   Establishing auditable guidelines
    – joint patient/professional working group which drew up basic standards for the consultation, and suggested the introduction of a patient information leaflet
    – converting the standards into auditable guidelines
    – designing the audit procedure
    – designing the patient information leaflet

3   Piloting and auditing the guidelines and use of the leaflet
    – working with hospital management on an organisational level
    – working with consultants/teams to implement and audit the guidelines

The first two stages proved comparatively simple, although there were logistical problems both in making appointments to see consultants and in arranging mutually acceptable times for meetings of the joint working group. A set of basic, measurable guidelines embracing both organisation and communication was drawn up. While these would not ensure an ideal interview, they should prevent major problems.

The guidelines were adopted enthusiastically by one medical team, and an evaluation of their use is under way using interviews with patients. A second team is also currently looking into the integration of the guidelines into patient-centred care. This is being piloted at one of the participating hospitals. No significant problems were identified with either the guidelines themselves or with the procedure established for auditing them in outpatient departments. These guidelines* were published in May 1996 and are available from the King's Fund.

However, the pilot and audit were prevented from taking place in a number of areas, partly because of major changes in progress at the three hospitals, and also because of a series of minor organisational problems. Individually, these would appear trivial, but they combined to make implementation impossible at that time.

A number of suggestions were made both for future training of doctors and for the involvement of trained volunteers in providing information and support at the time of diagnosis.

The study demonstrated that problems in communication can be addressed, at least in part, by basic, measurable guidelines which require no special training to carry out. Although designed for use with cancer patients, they are adaptable to any other situation in which bad news has to be broken.

This model for joint patient/professional working could also be used in other areas where mutually acceptable solutions are needed to solve a jointly agreed problem.

---

* *Breaking Bad News. Guidelines and Patient Information Card.* Researched by the Patient Involvement Unit, Lynda Jackson Macmillan Centre for Cancer Support and Information, Mount Vernon Hospital and produced jointly with the King's Fund. 1996

Chapter 1

Introduction

The consultation at which patients are told that they have cancer is a major area of concern for both patients and health care staff and should be considered within the wider context of communication between hospitals and patients.

This study developed a new approach to improving the procedure for giving the cancer diagnosis and tested a model for involving patients and staff in the development of local cancer services. Qualitative research methods were used to obtain detailed information about their views and experiences, on the basis of which auditable guidelines for practice were established.

The project had the following aims:

- to find out what both patients and doctors consider to be the important elements of giving the cancer diagnosis, and how this might be improved
- to develop a set of guidelines based on the priorities established by this consultative exercise
- to use the guidelines to establish an auditable procedure for giving the cancer diagnosis which is acceptable to patients and doctors
- to evaluate the effectiveness of this method of patient consultation and participation.

The setting

Mount Vernon Centre for Cancer Treatment serves a catchment area covering parts of Buckinghamshire, Berkshire, Hertfordshire, North London and Bedfordshire, with a population of approximately two million people. It is sited within a district general hospital, which, since the project began, has merged with Watford General Hospital to become the Mount Vernon and Watford Hospitals NHS Trust. Consultant oncologists (cancer specialists) based at the Centre run clinics at 12 district general hospitals in the region. Interaction with staff in these hospitals enables the Centre to influence cancer care throughout its catchment area.

The project was carried out by staff of the Lynda Jackson Macmillan Centre for Cancer Support and Information, which opened in the grounds of the hospital in 1993. Staff from the centre have been pioneering methods of involving patients and health care staff both in setting research targets and in developing ways of working together. One of their aims is to develop and test a model for patient-centred care which would enable cancer services to be reviewed and improved systematically throughout the area.

The re-organisation of cancer services outlined in the Calman Report was announced after the project began. The Report proposes a three-tier system, with a cancer centre interacting with cancer units and primary care teams, based on a patient-centred approach.[1] This appears to offer an excellent opportunity for the implementation of a model for changing practice, such as that proposed for this study.

Involving local patient groups

An infrastructure was already in place for involving patients in setting research priorities, using the network of local community-based cancer support groups established over the past four years. An initial mapping exercise had identified 18 cancer support groups in the catchment area.[2] Links were established with the groups, and a directory was produced. Regular network days now take place, at which members come together to discuss topics of concern and to exchange ideas. In addition, representatives from the groups and health care staff from both hospital and community met regularly as a liaison group over a period of two years. Discussion of issues at this forum helped to promote mutual understanding, and provided experience of joint staff/patient working.[3]

Project design

Although communication skills training has been shown to be effective,[4] the persistence of problems with communication convinced the research team that an alternative approach was required. Initial discussions suggested that an effective way to change the practice of professionals giving the diagnosis might be to establish an auditable procedure. This would consist of simple guidelines concerning the way the diagnosis should be given. The use of auditable standards would bring communication into line with procedures such as biopsy and wound dressing, thereby increasing its perceived status.

The second decision, based on previous work undertaken with the liaison group, was that input into the project should come from both doctors who gave the cancer diagnosis and patients who received it, so that the problems experienced by both parties to the communication could be addressed in establishing the guidelines.

It was also decided that the methods used in the data-gathering stages of the project should be based on a qualitative approach developed by the College of Health in seeking consumer views of the health service.[5] This would provide detailed information about the views and experiences of both patients and doctors, on which the guidelines could be based.

The three-stage process used to carry out the project is outlined in Figure 1 and discussed in more detail below.

Stage 1	Data gathering	Literature review Review of current practice Feedback from patients – 4 focus groups – 10 semi-structured interviews Feedback from doctors – 27 semi-structured interviews
Stage 2	Establishing auditable guidelines	Joint working group Putting the guidelines into auditable form Designing the intervention Designing the audit process
Stage 3	Piloting and auditing the guidelines	Working with hospital management Working with individual consultants

Figure 1 The three stages of the project

Choice of feedback methods

Patients' views and experiences were sought through both focus groups and semi-structured interviews. In obtaining feedback from doctors, however, individual interviews were the method chosen, because it was felt that doctors would feel more able to express doubt and uncertainty in an individual interview than in a group.

In all cases an interview schedule rather than a questionnaire was used so that the respondents could set out their own priorities rather than respond to a pre-set agenda.

Chapter 2

Stage 1: Data gathering

Review of the literature

Communication between doctor and patient has been the subject of much research in recent years, and yet evidence persists of patient dissatisfaction.[6] As patients seek to be more fully informed about their condition and involved in decisions about their care, they expect and demand improved communication skills from their doctors.[7] Concern over the way the cancer diagnosis is communicated has arisen because of the potential long-term effects upon patients; many feel that the communication has been handled badly at the start not only of their experience of hospital care but also of their personal struggle with the disease.

The inclusion of communication skills training in the medical curriculum is recommended by the General Medical Council but is not a requirement; and evidence suggests that it is not always accorded sufficient emphasis in medical schools. In some, less than 5 per cent of training time is spent on interpersonal skills, which are frequently not assessed formally.[8] Other studies indicate that doctors need to improve their communication skills [9] and that although the majority of bad news interviews take place in hospitals,[10] assessment of interpersonal communication skills using rating scales has been developed largely in association with the training of GPs rather than hospital doctors.[11,12,13]

Doctors tend to be worse at listening to patients when discussing psychosocial rather than medical topics, and even after training young doctors remain less effective at discussing such topics.[14]

Research into communication of the cancer diagnosis has highlighted the complexity of conveying information of an emotionally charged nature to patients.[15] Studies have shown that doctors' fear of difficult questions or of unleashing powerful emotions leads to distancing techniques which can result in selective attention, failure to follow up emotional cues, or giving false reassurance.[16,17]

The recognition of the importance of communication skills in this area has resulted in specially designed training courses and information on how best to organise and prepare for giving bad news. Studies of the effect of training on competence have shown that the improvement is a lasting one which cannot be matched simply by increased experience.[18]

Communication is a two-way process. While research among doctors has concentrated on their ability to communicate and on the development of interventions to improve these skills, patient research has concentrated on how much patients retain of what is communicated in the interview, rather than on how it is communicated. Giving an audiotape of the consultation is one way of overcoming the fact that shock may affect recall of what was communicated. However, while patients appreciate the chance to listen to the tapes[19] there is evidence that in cases where prognosis is poor the giving of the tape may increase psychological morbidity.[20]

There have been few studies of users' preferences in the communication of bad news. A detailed study into the experiences of parents who had been given the diagnosis of a life-threatening illness in their children showed that the quality of the bad news interview had affected subsequent ability to cope with the illness. Researchers commented on the vividness with which respondents were able to recall that interview, even many years afterwards.[21]

Review of current practice

For the majority of patients, the first stage in their experience of cancer is the visit to the GP with symptoms which may or may not suggest to the doctor the possibility of cancer. The patient will then probably be referred on to a consultant's outpatient clinic for investigations. The appointment is usually sent to the patient by post.

At the first consultation, the patient's medical history is taken and an examination carried out. The consultant may, at this stage, be more or less certain of the diagnosis, but will usually request further investigations. Tests such as scans, X-rays and blood tests are generally done on an outpatient basis, but the patient may have to be admitted to hospital for more invasive tests such as biopsy or laparotomy.

The results of outpatient or minimally invasive inpatient tests will be given at a further outpatient consultation. If a major operation such as a bowel resection has been required, the results will be given on the ward and are sent directly there.

A significant number of patients, however, do not follow this route. They may:

- be admitted as emergencies
- have their cancer diagnosed during investigation or treatment of another condition
- be diagnosed as a result of screening programmes.

The route taken and the amount of preparation the patients receive will inevitably affect their reception of the diagnosis.

Outpatient departments are generally able to identify by the beginning of a clinic which patients will be receiving results which could be considered 'bad news'. Results of investigations are sent to the consultant's secretary, who arranges for the consultant to read and sign them. In the departments of surgery and medicine at Mount Vernon, the results are separated at this stage into those which are considered 'routine' and those which give cause for concern. The former are filed in the patient's medical notes, and the latter are held separately in a clip and taken across to the clinic where they are read by the nurse in charge, who can then alert both the doctor and any support services which may be available. In plastic surgery outpatients at Mount Vernon and at Watford, the results are not specifically separated in this way, but the clinic nurses and doctors are able to read the results in advance and so prepare for the interview.

The system on the wards is less clear cut. Results of investigations arrive at intervals during the day, and are sometimes given by telephone. They eventually arrive on the junior doctor's desk, but there is no standard route by which they reach it.

Feedback from patients

This section examines the issues raised and experiences described when people affected by cancer were asked how they were given the diagnosis. For many, they were describing a critical event in their lives – one which they remembered clearly even though it had happened several years before. Some remembered it with tears, some philosophically and some with anger. Recounting experiences with the benefit of hindsight may not present an accurate view of what actually occurred. However it does offer a 'patient perspective' which has validity for the individual, and it is individual views which form the basis of this research.

Focus groups

Focus groups* were held with four cancer support groups. These were geographically spread over the catchment area of Mount Vernon Centre for Cancer Treatment and would use different District General Hospitals. One was a group for women with breast cancer, and the others included members with any cancer diagnosis. All welcomed relatives and friends.

Representatives from all the local groups formed a cancer support group network committee, and they discussed the topic at a special meeting. They had been asked to collect information from their group members and come to the meeting prepared to suggest guidelines. In order to see if the support group members expressed views which differed from other patient groups, a focus group was also held with patients who regularly attended a relaxation class at the Lynda Jackson Macmillan Centre.

Each group was asked to give views on how giving the cancer diagnosis could be improved. The discussion was tape-recorded, transcribed and the information analysed in order to identify the most important issues for patients and what guidelines they would recommend.

In-depth semi-structured interviews

Ten in-depth interviews were carried out with patients who at the time were attending an oncology outpatient clinic at Mount Vernon. The sample was randomly selected from a clinic list, and letters asking for the patients' consent to take part were handed out at the end of their appointment. Fourteen agreed to take part (of whom ten were selected for interview), five refused and ten did not reply. Interviews were carried either at the patient's home, or in the Lynda Jackson Macmillan Centre or by telephone, at the patient's choice.

---

* A focus group is a group, usually of between seven and twelve people, which is convened to discuss specific issues in an informal way in order to identify areas of mutual interest or concern.

These patients had different diagnoses, and although all had continued to receive follow-up care, the date of the original diagnosis varied from one to 13 years earlier. While cancer care has changed over that period and this might have made some of their experiences 'out of date', the profile of this group closely resembled the profile of support group members. All the individual patients interviewed had been given the diagnosis by a surgeon: seven at an outpatient appointment and three as inpatients.

Comparison of different methods of collecting patient views

Time

Although focus groups were more time-consuming than individual interviews, (up to two hours as against one hour or less for telephone interviews), and also required more secretarial time (up to seven hours), the views of a number of people could be obtained in one session. They were thus a quicker method of gaining information.

Detail

Qualitative research relies on detailed information, and more detail about people's experience was obtained from individual interviews. Some members of the focus groups gave lengthy individual accounts of their experiences and described their feelings in an uninhibited way. However, in other larger groups, those who were less comfortable with each other showed more reticence in talking about what was a very personal experience.

Type of data

The research aimed to gain information upon which guidelines could be based, and both focus groups and individuals were asked to suggest guidelines. This requires objective and analytical skills, and proved a more difficult task than relating individual experiences, which patients seemed to find therapeutic. The Cancer Support Group Network Committee members already had experience of translating qualitative evidence into a strategy, and they were the most effective at producing guidelines. However, some individuals interviewed also made useful suggestions on the basis of their own experience. A comparison of the guidelines is shown in Figure 2, on page 14.

Support groups as representatives of the views of patients

Concern had been expressed about just how representative the focus groups would be of patients' views in general. It was felt that support groups attracted those who were disaffected towards the medical profession, and might therefore express comparatively negative views. Comparison between the experiences related by the relaxation group and support groups indicated that members of the relaxation group had at least as many, if not more negative perceptions. However, support group members were more likely than non-members to think badly of their doctor when things went wrong. The evidence suggested that while both the group members and individual patients interviewed had experiences to complain about, group members were more likely do so.

When the purpose of the exercise is to identify areas where practice can be improved and not to evaluate a service, canvassing the views of support groups can be a useful exercise, because members are used to talking openly about cancer and exchanging ideas.

When guidelines are needed, the experienced group members who represent their members' views and can be objective about personal data, help to create a bridge between patients and doctors.

Findings

These findings are based on the key issues which emerged from the focus groups and individual interviews. Patients saw the bad news interview as just one part of their 'patient journey'. The events and feelings which led up to the interview had a bearing on how they experienced that interview, and what happened in the interview could affect how they subsequently coped with having cancer.

The issues below give a broad overview of the patient perspective from which guidelines can be developed. Detailed supporting quotations from patients are given in Appendix 1.

Preparation

The main cause of distress for patients was the shock of being told that they had cancer, which was associated in their minds both with an early and unexpected end to life and with unpleasant treatments.

Some said that it had been more of a shock because they were completely unprepared for 'bad news'; a number of factors had led patients to believe there was little to worry about, including:

- initial tests which were negative or routine
- being young and healthy
- false reassurance (however well intentioned) from friends, relatives, and sometimes GPs.

While some GPs were obviously aware that preparation was useful, patients indicated that others were so low key about the referral that the patient failed to appreciate how serious it might be.

In spite of all the clues to the contrary, some patients said that they never suspected it was cancer. One way of coping with the anxiety may well have been not to admit to oneself the truth, and some felt that not suspecting beforehand had saved them a lot of anxiety.

However, being already prepared for the diagnosis meant that, although it could still be a shock, it was less of one; preparation and honesty did seem to improve the experience.

It was felt that clearer language might have helped towards a realisation of the seriousness of the condition. One patient said that she suspected that the doctors had known it might be serious because she had heard one of them remark later that, when they operated, it was not as bad as expected.

The prior knowledge of their condition that patients bring to the diagnosis interview clearly has a bearing on how the news is received. Feedback from this study indicates that preparation for bad news lessens the impact. The GP and the specialist could both have a role to play in preparing the patient, and this may require closer liaison between the two. Concerns have been expressed that more information at this early stage might increase the patient's anxiety, perhaps unnecessarily, and if patients choose to 'deny' obvious signs and signals, this way of coping should be respected. However, the findings suggest that honest but sensitive preparation could help the patient in the diagnosis interview.

Doctors' manner/attitude

The attitude of the doctor breaking the bad news was important to patients. They spoke positively of doctors who were confident, positive, matter of fact, caring and honest. A number of people emphasised the importance of the doctor telling them the truth and some suggested that doctors were themselves afraid to use the word 'cancer'. However, while some patients said that they preferred a straightforward approach, others complained of doctors being too blunt.

Doctors in the past seem to have taken the attitude that diagnosis is merely a question of giving a medical opinion, but this left some patients quite devastated. The doctor's attitude could make the world of difference to cancer patients; what was most appreciated was a caring, human manner which lacked arrogance.

Finding an approach which suits each patient is clearly difficult. Some felt it should be clear cut and to the point, others felt that they would prefer a more gentle and circumspect approach to the subject. The difficulty for many doctors giving the diagnosis is that they may not know the patient very well, if at all. Judging how to deliver the news to that individual then becomes almost impossible, and doctors are bound occasionally to strike the wrong note.

Lack of rapport

Patients explained how difficult they found the interview because they did not know the doctor, and this was worse when the doctor failed to introduce him or herself. The interview was seen as the beginning of a crucial relationship which would continue throughout treatment. At the same time it was recognised that the doctor faced a very difficult task in breaking the bad news to someone they do not know, and that they might adopt a standard information-giving approach when faced with this task.

Being told by someone they already knew did seem to make a considerable difference to some, and this gave rise to discussion in the groups about who might be the best person to give the cancer diagnosis. Members were divided over the respective merits of having a doctor who knows the patient or a specialist in the disease. There seemed to be no hard-and-fast rule. Some people got on well with their GPs and would have preferred to hear the diagnosis from them; others did not. There would be practical problems as well as a need for clarification of roles if someone other than the specialist gave the diagnosis. Communicating such important information when there is no pre-existing relationship clearly presents difficulties to both doctor and patient.

Language

Many people referred to the fact that the word 'cancer' was not used initially in the interview, and that this led to uncertainty about the nature of the diagnosis. Some patients felt that it was not only the patient's fear that was a barrier to clear communication, but also the doctor's. However, there were also some patients who did not like the use of the word 'cancer' and took some time to adjust to its use in relation to themselves.

The use of long or complicated medical terms also confused people. Those who were diagnosed with a pre-cancerous conditions found it particularly difficult to understand the nature of their diagnosis. Clear language, sensitively used, helped patients to understand, and gave them more sense of control over the situation. Although some patients reacted quite strongly against the use of the word 'cancer', these retrospective views suggest that many others would like the diagnosis of cancer to be clearly stated at the start.

Having someone with you

Not everyone wanted a relative or friend with them at the diagnosis interview. However others felt strongly that they would have liked someone with them and that they had to cope with the shock and confusion unsupported. Supportive friends or relatives were seen as important for two principal reasons. First, that while the patient went into shock on hearing the diagnosis, the supporter could act as the 'ears' of the patient, and ask key questions. Second, the patient was often in such a state of shock following the interview that they required assistance with getting home. The key role of the family in supporting the patient was apparent from many of the accounts, and providing an opportunity for them to be involved from the early stages was obviously a healing process in itself.

Group members felt that patients should be offered the choice of having their partner with them at the diagnosis interview, and that if the patient chose to be told alone, the doctor should offer to go through the diagnosis again with the relative present. Of course, this can only be an option if a relative has accompanied the patient to the interview; often the patient had not thought to bring anyone. It was suggested that patients should be advised by their GP or specialist to bring someone with them, or that staff could phone a relative and ask them to come to the hospital. When someone needed support during and after the interview and a relative or friend was not there, it was felt to be important that the support of a specialist nurse was offered.

It is difficult to find ways of empowering patients in this situation when they themselves are so vulnerable, but having an 'advocate', be it relative, friend, counsellor or volunteer, can be one way of doing so.

The needs of relatives

Involving relatives at the diagnosis stage can also highlight their need for information and support. Some patients said that their partner did not know what questions to ask in the consultation, and others complained about not having been given enough information. There appeared to be inconsistencies in the way in which relatives were involved at the diagnosis stage, and it was strongly suggested that a consistent approach should be adopted. Accounts indicated that when relatives were told separately, this could set up barriers between patient and relative. Some patients found telling the news to their partner a heavy burden, and others felt that relatives should not be able to prevent the patient's knowing their diagnosis, as this also could set up barriers. A relative's view of the ideal situation is given in Appendix 1.

Involving relatives in receiving the 'bad news' presents a number of difficulties for the health professional. He or she must first discover to what extent the patient wishes them to be involved. Some patients preferred that their spouse was not present or saw it as an additional burden. However, relatives or carers have their own needs. A study of the views of carers undertaken in Hillingdon (available from the authors) showed that carers are at least as anxious as the patient, and often more so. Ways need to be found of meeting the information and support needs of carers, whether they are told with the patient or at some other time.

Support

Many patients were extremely traumatised following the bad news interview and thought that information about sources of support should be given at the interview so that patients and relatives could obtain help later when they wanted it. When a specialist nurse was present at the interview and talked to the patient afterwards, this seemed to be very useful, and many patients felt that there should be counsellors or specialist nurses available in every hospital. However, not everyone took up the offer of continued support. Some patients felt it was unnecessary and some that there had been a lack of rapport, while others found it difficult to take in what was said.

Patients used different sources of support: their GP, a nurse on the ward, colleagues at work, voluntary organisations such as BACUP and Breast Cancer Care. Several said that they would have liked to have spoken to someone with a similar diagnosis. The kind of support patients looked for afterwards was associated with emotional and practical aspects of having the disease, aspects which patients often did not expect to discuss with specialists whom they saw as dealing with diagnosis and treatment. Members of one of the groups said that they would have liked more contact with their GP following diagnosis.

In order to find support following diagnosis patients need information about sources and choices. It is still a matter of luck whether patients receive written information about voluntary support groups and organisations or whether they are told about specialist nurses. The *Coping with Your Cancer* [22] and *Help Is There* [23] leaflets are both designed to give this kind of information. Methods of ensuring that this information reaches the patient need to be found. Many patients spoke of 'just being left', and although this is less common with the introduction of specialist nurses, it remains a major issue for those who did not receive this kind of help. This clearly has implications for staffing, and may require the re-examination of professional roles.

Other things happening in people's lives

Of the ten patients interviewed, five mentioned other difficulties which they had to cope with at the time of their cancer diagnosis. For example, one woman's husband was having his third hip replacement operation, two patients had recently lost a parent, and one had three young children, one of whom was disabled. It was therefore important that patients were asked what other difficulties they might be experiencing and were given information about where to get further support.

Information, treatment and choice

Many patients said that after they were given the diagnosis they could not take in anything which was said to them. Several ideas were suggested to overcome this, including:

- giving written information
- tape-recording the interview
- having a relative or friend present.

Patients spoke of needing time to pull themselves together and to get over the shock, but then to have an opportunity to ask questions in order to allay their fears. Some said that they should be invited to return the next day, when they had recovered from the shock, to ask questions and discuss treatment plans.

A positive message

Patients' information needs included a clear diagnosis and a treatment plan, which was important so that they felt there was something which could be done. Giving a positive message was thought to be very important. Some patients wanted to hear about treatment options at the diagnosis interview, and others very soon afterwards. They also wanted information about the process, about what was going to happen, and about choices. The importance of allowing time to make decisions was emphasised. Some patients felt very bitter about decisions which had been made hastily or without their involvement.

Those who complained most vociferously about lack of information had been diagnosed some years previously, and it is clear that patients are now being given more information. They are also, as a result of media coverage, expecting more information from medical staff. Individual patients and carers had different information needs, but there was general agreement that they would like more, and that information was closely associated both with a sense of control and with feeling positive. When patients are in a state of shock they may not take in information, and so ways of obtaining it need to be flexible and easily accessible.

Privacy/vulnerability

People given the cancer diagnosis on the ward while they were in bed commented on the lack of privacy. Even when the curtains were drawn around the bed, the conversation could be heard by other patients, and there was nowhere private to come to terms with the news. However, while the ward lacked privacy, it could offer a source of support.

Lack of privacy, and the fact that the patient is in bed and may be quite ill mean that he or she may feel vulnerable. Being told when lying down and being in a state of undress (which was felt to be an embarrassing and difficult experience at any time) also contributed to this feeling of vulnerability.

Ensuring privacy in an outpatient department may be straightforward, although even there, patients sometimes have to walk out of the consulting room in distress into a waiting room full of other patients. Finding ways of avoiding this – for example, by the doctor leaving the patient in the room to recover – would be helpful. When patients are told on the ward, ensuring privacy is more difficult, particularly where the patient is frail and confined to bed. However, there may be ways in which other patients could be prevented from overhearing, and these should be considered.

Time

It is interesting to note the issues which were not raised in this study. Very few patients referred to whether or not they had had enough time in the interview, although some said that they had had no sense of time because of the impact of the diagnosis. Time was, however, a factor which patients felt affected the manner or attitude of the doctor giving the diagnosis.

This is probably a more obvious issue to doctors than to patients (see page 15). Allowing time may help the doctor to carry out the interview without additional stress, and this may well improve the communication. Finding ways of achieving this is an organisational problem. However, as patients pointed out, the time does not have to be that of a busy consultant: it could be a support nurse.

When patients 'discover' their diagnosis

Not all patients found out that they had cancer through their doctor. A few described how they had found out by accident or deduced the diagnosis themselves. Group members also gave instances of patients who had been given the news over the telephone, which they felt was wrong as there might not be anyone there to offer support. Supporting patients who 'discover' their diagnosis requires a flexible approach through which support can be easily obtained.

Guidelines

The guidelines suggested by groups, individual patients and the network committee are shown in Figure 2 for purposes of comparison.

Discussion

Patients view the bad news interview as just one part of their cancer journey, but a crucial one. Getting the communication right for the patient is therefore an important, but not easy, task. The findings show that individual patients and relatives have different ways of coping and responding. Getting it right, especially where the doctor and patient may well not know each other, is asking a lot of both parties. However, the findings indicate that the attitude and communication skills of the doctor are very important, and that being aware of what individual patients bring to the interview, and what they will require afterwards is also vital.

This is not a situation in which it is easy to 'empower the patient', because it is a time when, faced with one's own mortality, one is in a most vulnerable state. However, it was suggested that the following can all help:

INDIVIDUALS (numbers suggesting guideline)	FOCUS GROUPS	NETWORK COMMITTEE	COMMITTEE COMMENTS
Should be prepared by doctor for news (3)	Give more information, especially in writing	Give information	Especially contact numbers for support and further information
Dr should be confident (1), positive (2) matter of fact (1)	Give a positive message	Maximise privacy	Use designated room. Pulling curtains is not enough
Ask patient what he/she thinks is wrong (1)	Patients should have someone with them	Patients need a supporter	Relative, friend or health professional
Explain treatment asap after diagnosis, allowing time for shock to subside (3)	Treatment should be explained	Give a positive message	Something can always be found. Avoid giving limits for life expectancy
Explain treatment options clearly (1)	Doctor should be caring	Be aware of sensitivity	Eye contact & body language. Easier if the patient is already known. Acknowledge feelings
Allow time for decisions about treatment (1)	Allow time for decisions	Allow patient to take one step at a time	Decisions may have to be delayed to allow time for thought. Follow-up appt made for this
Use clear language – cancer rather than malignancy or tumour	Use simple, non-medical language, and be honest	Use clear language	Check understanding. Explain medical terms. Offer interpreter – do not rely on family
Arrange nurse to talk to patient afterwards, especially if doctor is busy (3)	Arrange support afterwards	Avoid interruptions	Includes phone calls, reading notes without discussion & talking to colleagues
Give information re. sources of support, e.g. BACUP, support nurses	Doctor should plan the giving of the news	Avoid physical barriers	Includes desks, white coats etc
	Doctor should introduce himself	Patients should know whom they are speaking to & be addressed by name	All health professionals should introduce themselves & explain roles.
	Patient should be clothed	Patient deserves respect	Patient should be dressed and sitting up whenever possible
		Relatives have needs	Information and support

Figure 2 The guidelines suggested by patients

- having a relative, friend or counsellor present as advocate and supporter
- giving positive messages, using appropriate language and providing patients with the information they want
- giving details of sources of support and information

can all help.

Feedback from doctors

This section reviews the results obtained from interviews with 27 consultants, all of whom regularly have to tell patients that they have cancer. The interviews were intended to obtain both factual information and subjective opinions. (See Table 1 for a breakdown of the consultants' specialties.)

Table 1 Specialties of consultants interviewed, including one consultant in 2 specialties

General surgery	3	General medicine	3
Plastic surgery	4	Palliative medicine	2
Gastroenterology	2	Urology	1
Gynaecology	2	Geriatrics	2
ENT	3	Haematology	2
Oral surgery	1	Orthopaedics (incl. 1 A&E)	3

The majority of consultations in which bad news is given take place in hospital,[10] and since hospital services remain substantially consultant-led, the interest and co-operation of consultants concerned with cancer patients were a prerequisite. It was also hoped that the interviews would raise the general level of awareness of communication as a process which needs as much thought and preparation as other areas of clinical practice.

Selecting and contacting the doctors

All consultants at Mount Vernon and Watford General Hospitals who, at the time of the study, were involved in the diagnosis of new malignancies, were sent a letter asking them to participate in the study by agreeing to be interviewed by a researcher. Time constraints meant that only a proportion of consultants at each hospital could be interviewed, and the aim of the subsequent selection was to encompass as wide a range of specialties as possible, while maintaining an emphasis on those whose work brought them regularly into contact with cancer patients.

Making contact with some of the consultants proved to be a major hurdle for the research team. Although in many cases this was a straightforward process, it frequently involved far more phone calls (the record was nine) than had been expected. The protracted nature of this process could have serious implications for the cost of conducting such a study.

The interviews lasted an average of three-quarters of an hour, the shortest being 15 minutes and the longest one and a half hours. They ranged from simple, often one word answers to the questions in the schedule, to wide-ranging discussions in which the questions acted merely as a guide to areas of interest. In some cases a nurse or secretary was present and participated in the discussion.

The responses

The range of opinions on many of the questions was very wide, although several consultants told the interviewer that they assumed that the views of their colleagues would be very similar to their own. Supporting quotations are given in Appendix 2.

Estimated level of contact with newly diagnosed cancer patients

The consultants were asked to estimate how frequently they had to tell patients they had cancer; exact figures could have been found, but the aim of this question was to gauge how familiar a process it was for them. Estimates ranged from one per year from one of the orthopaedic surgeons to 200 per year from a plastic surgeon.

An orthopaedic surgeon who estimated that he saw very few initial diagnoses of cancer gave this as one of the main reasons for his choice of medical specialty, as he found the breaking of such news extremely distressing. In marked contrast was the plastic surgeon who saw several newly diagnosed cancer patients each week and felt that giving the diagnosis was simply one of the things that had to be done.

Because those interviewed were from a wide range of medical specialties, the types of cancer they encountered varied considerably, as did their frequency of occurrence. For some, such as orthopaedic surgeons, new primary cancers are a rare occurrence; they are more likely to be presented with bone metastases from a primary cancer the existence of which may or may not have been previously known. For others, the patients they see may regularly present with symptoms which arouse suspicion, and so the proportion of totally unprepared patients will be significantly lower.

Communication skills training

Consultants were asked both about their experience, if any, of such training and about whether they would attend such a course if one were offered which was designed specifically for consultants. Only two of the consultants had experienced formal communication skills training, mainly because such courses were not part of medical training when they were students. A number of those who had expressed a particular interest in doctor–patient communication said that this had been kindled by the experience of working with a charismatic consultant earlier in their careers. Indeed one consultant, who now spends many hours discussing treatments and their implications, had been on the verge of leaving medicine altogether before meeting the doctor whose enthusiasm and patience led to this conversion.

Despite their lack of experience of communication skills courses, and in the face of well documented success[4] most of those interviewed held very strong opinions about the value of such courses. The format of such training was also questioned, and it was generally felt that the best way to learn communication skills was by means of an 'apprenticeship', working with live situations rather than having didactic instruction.

Of those interviewed, five expressed a positive interest in such a course. Some were already actively engaged in training junior doctors and therefore understandably felt that they would not need any further training themselves, but would rather be involved in giving the training. The scepticism expressed in the replies to the question about experience of training was again apparent in the response to this question, and similar comments were made. The difficulty of fitting such a course into an already congested schedule was also pointed out; doctors felt that their time was better spent seeing patients in a clinic than at a training course.

Response to being interviewed

In many cases the interviews appeared to stimulate a previously unexplored interest in the process of communication, and many positive comments were made. Consultants seem to have ample opportunity for discussion of clinical issues, particularly where these involve new or unusual conditions and treatments. Other areas of their clinical practice appear to be talked about less regularly, if at all, and several of the respondents said that they had appreciated the chance to talk over the issues in an unthreatening and uninterrupted way. Once the time had been set aside for the interview, it became available for more far-reaching discussions than it is possible to do justice to in this report.

The sense of isolation mentioned earlier was highlighted by the following contrasting comments: 'Was I normal?' (Consultant A) and
'I expect everyone thinks the way I do.' (Consultant B). These consultants work together in the same department.

The bad news interview

This section summarises the responses given to questions directly concerned with the practicalities and content of the bad news interview.

Table 2 Where the news is broken

Mainly in outpatient dept	11	Could be either	12
Mainly on the ward	4		

For most consultants the setting for the bad news interview was not a matter of choice but depended on whether the patient needed to be admitted for investigations or other procedures. Those who were able to choose felt that it was easier to break the news on the ward, despite the problems arising from lack of privacy. Two of them made special arrangements for patients to be either brought or kept in specifically for that purpose. The reasons given were:

- it is easier to assess the patient's response
- ward staff are more used to dealing with emotional crises than clinic staff
- there is more opportunity to answer questions as they arise.

Many felt that a busy clinic was not the ideal place to be presenting people with such devastating news, and a few made special arrangements to see patients with a new diagnosis of cancer either before the main clinic or at the very end, when the pressure of time is not so great.

In some cases the physical layout of the clinic was such that patients making their way out of a bad news interview would necessarily have to walk through a long corridor past other waiting patients. The consultants working in these areas were fully aware that this was unsatisfactory, but recognised that it was beyond their control.

Table 3 Who gives the news

Always consultant except in emergency	11	Shared equally between the team	9
Consultant or senior colleague	8	Usually a junior member of the team	1

Here again there was a considerable degree of consensus that a senior member of the team should generally be responsible for giving patients the news; this was felt to be easier to achieve in the outpatient setting than on the ward. It was pointed out that patients who attend a small hospital with few consulting rooms have a greater chance of seeing the consultant than those who attend large clinics. Some consultants made it an absolute rule that only they should undertake this task, and one said that he would rather delegate the surgery than the communication of the diagnosis. Their reasons for this were that they felt that they took ultimate responsibility for the overall handling of the case, and that junior doctors might not have sufficient experience to deal comfortably with giving the news. However, the majority felt that this task could be adequately undertaken by registrars and senior registrars.

Several used their consultations with patients as an opportunity for teaching junior staff by example, and indeed many believed this to be the most effective means of learning about the communication of bad news. One felt the ability to teach in this way was an indication of the degree of competence of the consultant. Further discussion in this area revealed that some of these consultants had not considered the inherent weakness in this approach, which is that unsatisfactory performance by senior staff could lead to a perpetuation of their insensitive or inappropriate methods of communication.

Two consultants expressed concern about the conflict between their responsibility to patients and the need for junior staff to practise their communication skills in a live situation, particularly when the junior staff in question are perceived as being in need of training.

Who else is there

In the majority of cases another professional is present when patients are told their diagnosis. In the outpatient department this is generally the clinic nurse or health care assistant, and on the wards it tends to be the named nurse where possible. Reasons given for this were either patient-focused – to 'pick up the pieces' – or for the doctor's protection to avoid litigation. In some cases junior staff are also encouraged to observe or participate in the interview, either as part of their training or because they will be taking over the day-to-day management of the patient. Some patients also bring friends or relatives with them, and this was generally thought to be a good thing, as friends or relatives were often able to take in information which the patient was too shocked to absorb.

Table 4 Telling patients by telephone

| Never | 12 | Regularly | 1 |
| Occasionally | 14 | | |

The majority of consultants believed that patients should not be told their diagnosis over the telephone if at all possible. Those who never did so felt very strongly that this was a completely unacceptable practice. However, many felt that there were occasions on which it was the easiest option, and there was one consultant who regularly told patients their diagnoses over the telephone and could see no reason why this should be regarded as unusual or unsatisfactory.

The content of the interview

There was further consensus about the overall content of the bad news interview, most consultants believing that, in addition to the results of investigations, patients should be told what types of treatment are available, and what the plan is for future management of the disease. It was felt to be important for an optimistic note to be struck, and one consultant explained that although not all problems could be solved, patients should know that they would not be abandoned but supported through them.

There are some patients whose first line treatment is radiotherapy or chemotherapy, and who will therefore not be treated by the consultant who has diagnosed their condition. In these circumstances it may not be possible for this consultant to explain the treatment in any detail. Some consultants run joint clinics with an oncologist, at which such patients can be seen by both specialists, thus avoiding the anxiety generated by the delay involved in a further referral.

Process and preparation

The giving of the cancer diagnosis emerged from the analysis as part of a process rather than as a single experience, and the so-called bad news interview itself was seen as part of two interlocking processes, the diagnostic and the information giving. For the patient, the diagnostic process starts with the first consultation with his GP and continues through consultant referral and investigations until a diagnosis is arrived at.

Many of the consultants also saw the giving of the information about the diagnosis as a process rather than as an isolated episode. They felt that because of the shock experienced by being given the news, patients were often unable to take in the rest of the consultation, and that information should be given gradually, with time allowed for the patient to reflect before coming back for further questions to be answered.

There was a range of views about the extent to which these processes are linked, and about the stage at which the information-giving process may become part of the diagnostic process. For some conditions the presenting symptom may immediately indicate that a diagnosis of cancer is possible; in such cases it is likely either that patients themselves may have suspicions or that the GP may indicate the possible outcome of the specialist referral. Several consultants believed that it was important to give an indication of the possibility of cancer at the initial consultation in order to allow the patient time to come prepared for the follow-up interview, and some believed that patients would deduce the possibility of cancer from the tests they were to have.

However, this was by no means a unanimously held view, and those who disagreed felt strongly that such preparation was not helpful to patients, and could put them through perhaps three weeks of anxiety to no purpose.

In cases where there may be little to alert the GP or the consultant at a first examination to the possibility of cancer, the information-giving process can only begin when the results of investigations become known, and the diagnosis is sometimes as much of a surprise to the doctor as it is to the patient.

Written information

Very little written information was given out by the consultants interviewed, mainly because they felt that the medical situation was too complex for any one piece of written information to be suitable. Some said that they would like to give patients something in writing if they could find the appropriate leaflet, but many believed that imparting information at the right time and in the right way for each patient was a subtle process which would not be enhanced by written information.

One consultant, however, did provide information which was individually written – and drawn – during the consultation so that the patient had the correct diagnosis and treatment plan, to look at later and as a basis for future questions. Another wrote to each patient following the consultation, reminding them of what had been discussed and enclosing a copy of the letter sent to the GP.

Documentation

Although there was widespread acknowledgement of the importance of documentation, very few consultants felt that they performed as well in this area as they should. Some pleaded lack of time, others lack of secretarial assistance. The degree to which they document the bad news interview is shown in Table 5.

Table 5

In full	5	Only in case of dispute	1
Detailed letter to GP	6	Only if not telling patient diagnosis	1
Less than they would like	11	Nothing written in notes	3

The experience of giving the cancer diagnosis

This section concentrates on the subjective responses given by consultants when asked about their personal experience of telling patients that they have cancer. The difficulties they described are outlined, together with some of the organisational and psychological barriers to effective communication.

There was little disagreement among those interviewed about the overall importance of the consultation in which the cancer diagnosis is given, although some doctors felt that other medical conditions were equally traumatic for patients to hear about, and that the importance of cancer was overplayed both in the media and by oncologists. However, opinion on the degree of priority which should be given to this part of the clinical process varied widely. There were those who regarded it as probably the most important aspect of their work, and felt that the whole future course of treatment was determined by how this interview was handled. A few felt that it was simply part of the job and should be done, as everything else should be done, as well as possible, and one said that although it was obviously important for the patient, it was of no particular significance to him.

Many consultants acknowledged that giving a patient the news that they have cancer was an inherently difficult area of their work, and although some felt that it was generally a difficult area rather than something which they personally had problems with, others said that they regularly found the experience distressing. The most extreme case was that of a consultant who had not slept for two nights the last time he had given a cancer diagnosis.

The specific difficulties mentioned included:

- **cancers** which are:
    - unexpected by the patient
    - unexpected by the doctor
    - difficult or impossible to treat
    - painful, disfiguring, or 'gruesome'

- **patients or relatives** who:
    - are angry, violent or distressed
    - demand what doctors perceive as excessive time or emotional support
    - do not wish their relatives to be told the truth
    - have major family responsibilities, especially parents of young children
    - are very young.

Of these, the angry or distressed patient or relative seemed to be the cause of the greatest problems for doctors, who either find it difficult to know how to respond to extremes of emotion, or feel under pressure to move patients through the consulting room quickly.

Another major problem is caused by the wish that many relatives have to protect the patient from the bad news; the tradition of telling relatives the diagnosis first is less widespread than it was, but in many cases they suspect that the patient may have cancer and feel that he or she will not be able to cope with the news. One consultant clearly felt that pressure from relatives to withhold information from the patient was a major source of difficulty.

Several comments were made on the influence of the media, whose widespread reporting of such issues as breast cancer was felt to have led to an excessive demand for information and choice from some patients.

There were few specific situations in which doctors found it easier to tell patients that they have cancer, although it was generally felt that patients who were prepared for the diagnosis, or who actually asked whether it was cancer, were less likely to become very distressed.

The response to the question about confidence in this area of work provided some interesting insights. Several of those who most regularly see new cancer patients expressed a surprising degree of diffidence about their own performance, and yet others who are very eminent in their field felt that they were more confident about communication than they were about their other clinical work. The researchers had wondered whether any link would be seen between confidence and frequency of breaking the bad news, but this was not by any means the case. It was pointed out that this area of work was one in which there was little opportunity for peer group support or discussion.

Barriers to good communication

The principal barriers identified by the consultants are examined below.

Time

Most of the consultants felt that lack of time, particularly in outpatient clinics, was the main reason why they were not able to communicate the bad news as effectively as they would like to. One surgeon, however, said that giving enough time was sufficiently important for him to *make* that time within the clinic setting, even if it meant that other patients had to wait longer. Others arranged their clinics in such a way that those whose results were expected to indicate a diagnosis of cancer were seen either before the clinic (some as early as 8am) or at the end of the clinic when there are no other patients to be kept waiting.

Lack of knowledge of the patient

The majority of patients who come for investigations will be unknown to the doctor before the first consultation, and there is little opportunity for the doctor to establish a rapport or to find out the patient's family background, beliefs and level of understanding, all of which will have an effect on the way in which the news of the diagnosis is received.

Problems of comprehension

There can be several reasons why patients fail to comprehend what the doctor is trying to tell them:

- English is not their first language
- they are too shocked to hear what is said
- the doctor uses medical jargon or ambiguous language.

The impact of the shock of the diagnosis was acknowledged by many doctors.

Guidelines and the use of audit

The range of opinion about the concept of auditable guidelines for the giving of the cancer diagnosis was very wide indeed.

- Some consultants were clearly resistant to the suggestion, and felt that their clinical independence might be compromised, although one did concede that there were times when guidelines were necessary.
- Some felt that such guidelines would have been very helpful to them when they were less experienced, and would be useful for teaching junior staff.
- Some believed very strongly in them.

They were, on the whole, interested in the idea of thinking about communication as a process to be analysed, and several said that they had never considered it in this way before.

The suggested guidelines

Some consultants, who clearly *had* thought about communication as a process, were able to suggest up to ten guidelines for the breaking of bad news without pausing for thought. Others, who had said that they did not approve of the concept of guidelines, nonetheless conceded that the answers they had given to earlier questions such as 'Who gives the news?' or 'Is the diagnosis ever given over the telephone?' did in fact amount to unwritten guidelines.

The most commonly suggested guidelines to emerge from the analysis fell into two main categories, namely organisational and communications-based, and are shown in Figure 3.

Discussion

The responses to the interviews outlined above show that consultants in a wide range of medical specialties are involved in telling patients that they have cancer. Many of them find this a difficult and demanding task, and they are far from unanimous both about whether patients should in principle be made fully aware of the situation and about how this is best done. There is ample evidence that, on the whole, patients prefer to be given information about their condition, and yet the myth persists that many do not wish to hear the news. There must clearly be scope for clinical judgement in this matter, as there will be occasions when it is not appropriate for patients to know their diagnosis, but work needs to be done in overcoming resistance to seeing information-giving as the norm rather than the exception.

How this can be achieved is a matter for debate. Consultants' attitudes to formal communication skills training are at best sceptical. Many seem to believe that this is an area of work in which ability is innate and cannot be improved upon. Those who believe that improvements *can* be made see little value in formal courses, believing rather that observation and supervised practice early in a doctor's career are the way forward.

ORGANISATION	COMMENTS	COMMUNICATION	COMMENTS
Allow time for patient to absorb news & ask questions (A)	Some consultants regard this as impossible	**Give a positive message (D)**	Mentioned by 13 consultants. May only mean patient knows he/she will not be abandoned
Give an opportunity for answering further questions	e.g. offer 2nd appointment, suggest phoning later	**Avoid lies & secrets (E,F)**	Includes ensuring everyone is told the same story
News to be given by senior team member	Not mentioned specifically, but a personal guideline for many	**Relate to patient's perspective**	Ask his/her view of situation and any specific anxieties
Patient sitting up & dressed (B)	Not always possible on ward; should be routine in outpatients, though 1 doctor disagreed.	**Give impression of time, never hurry (G)**	Concentrate on the patient, speak & act without haste, avoid interruptions
Maximise privacy (C)	Easier in outpatients, usually possible on ward, though not always done (A)	**Use simple language (H)**	Explain even simple medical terminology, Patients will not necessarily ask
Minimise disturbance	eg divert phone, give bleep to another team member	**Ensure that everyone uses the same language**	Many thought this important, but very few documented the language used
Have another professional present	Support nurse preferable. Suggested by some only to avoid litigation.	**Create confidence**	Not often suggested as guideline, more often mentioned in terms of professional relationship
Plan the interview	i.e. read results, be confident of diagnosis, think about future management		
Avoid talking across the desk	Opinions divided; some regarded this as completely unimportant		
Arrange support for giver of news **Have tissues available** **Arrange somewhere for patient to go to recover**	Each suggested by only one consultant	**Work up to it gradually** **Remember that silence is all right** **Let the patient know you find it difficult** **Always act (theatrically)** **Make physical contact**	Each suggested by only one consultant

Figure 3 The guidelines suggested by the consultants (references to supporting quotations, Appendix 1)

However, in the light of some areas of current practice, there must be doubt as to the example being given to the present generation of junior doctors, who will become the teachers of the future.

Chapter 2

Stage 2: Establishing auditable guidelines

Joint working group of health professionals and patient representatives

The group was set up to review the research reports on the patients' and doctors' views and to draw up guidelines for giving the cancer diagnosis. It comprised two surgeons, a specialist nurse, a counsellor, a facilitator, an oncologist, a GP and four patient representatives, who were recruited through the cancer support groups and included one person with experience as a carer.

The group was facilitated in a structured way so that the task could be completed as efficiently as possible; staff taking part in a previous joint patient/health professional group had commented that the lack of formal structure led to time being wasted.[3] All members had an opportunity to read the reports, but the researchers presented the group with a list of the key points raised by doctors and patients from which to draw up the guidelines. There were four meetings. At the first, the group agreed a way of working together and had preliminary discussion of the reports. The second meeting identified those elements of the bad news interview without which it would not be satisfactory, and also the interventions necessary and how these could be evaluated. At the third, the guidelines were agreed and ways of implementing them discussed.

A further meeting was held six months later to discuss progress in the implementation of the guidelines.

The guidelines as drawn up by the group

> **Referral** from GP to the specialist should include information about the patient, and the GP should explain to the patient what to expect.
>
> **Prior to the consultation** the **specialist** requires a precise diagnosis where possible, a family history, and knowledge of the patient's understanding of their disease. Preparation time is also required.
>
> **Prior to the consultation** the **patient** requires waiting times in clinic to be minimised, and to be told that they can bring a friend or relative.
>
> **During the consultation** the **specialist** requires a quiet, private and uninterrupted environment, a support nurse, time, and the patient in as good a condition to receive the news as possible (e.g. sitting up and dressed).
>
> **During the consultation** the **patient** requires the doctor to introduce him/herself and the support nurse, address them by their name, make eye contact, and give a message of hope.
>
> **Throughout the interview** the **specialist** should check that the patient understands, and by the end of the interview the patient should have as clear an idea as possible of what the diagnosis is. Information given about future treatment should be explained, including the physical sensations to be expected. Personalised written information should be given which includes:

– the name of the specialist and support nurse together with contact details
– where to get further support and information
– the date of the next appointment.

A general information leaflet about the condition should also be given.

After the consultation the **specialist** should ensure that a support nurse is available and that appropriate arrangements have been made for returning home, follow-up support, tests, appointments and the needs of relatives.

After the consultation the **specialist** should send information to the GP which includes the name of the support nurse, what was said in the consultation and how it was received.

Suggestions made by the group to complement the guidelines

The group identified gaps in communication between the patient's GP and the hospital, both at the referral stage and when the diagnosis had been made. In order to bridge this gap two interventions were suggested.

- A referral form on which the GP could communicate relevant information about the patient being referred, including information about what prompted the GP to refer the patient and about what the patient should expect from the hospital appointment. This would also advise patients of their right to bring a relative to the consultation.
- A form giving details of the bad news interview to be sent to the patient's GP.

Because patients often could not remember the details of the diagnosis interview as a result of shock at hearing the news, a patient information sheet was also proposed. This would be filled in by the person giving the diagnosis, and would include:

- details of the patient's condition
- whom they had seen
- what would happen next
- whom they could contact for support and information.

It would then be given to the patient to take home.

Advantages and disadvantages of using the group

Advantages

- Patient representatives and health professionals were able to put across their views and seek mutually agreed solutions. In fact there was considerable common ground. Supporting quotations from group members are given in Appendix 3.

- Health professionals had a thorough knowledge of current systems and procedures, and were therefore able to suggest ideas which would be practical and acceptable to colleagues.

- Patient representatives were able to offer a different perspective on priorities and difficulties.

- Interaction between the two perspectives brought about a better understanding of the issues, and was a learning experience in itself.

- Professionals were able to identify gaps in communication and differences in procedures.

Disadvantages

- Difficulty of arranging a suitable time for all members of the group

- Difficulty of ensuring a stable group. One of the patient representatives withdrew because of illness and another died (neither as a result of cancer). This left the group balanced in favour of the professional perspective.

- With only four meetings, members had little opportunity to establish a rapport, which takes longer in a mixed group.

- The doctors tended to dominate the discussion initially, and careful facilitation was needed to ensure that the patient representatives had an opportunity to put across their points. After the initial meeting the facilitator had a separate meeting with the patient representatives to encourage them to work out and articulate what they wished to say.

The audit process

Putting the guidelines into auditable form

The guidelines as drawn up by the group took the form of a series of requirements for a successful consultation. These had then to be written in a way which would allow their implementation to be audited. The researchers were given helpful advice by the Clinical Audit Department at Mount Vernon and Watford Hospitals NHS Trust, who also assisted in the production of an audit form (Appendix 4). The form was designed to be completed partly by the consultant and partly by the clinic nurse, and was checked for practicability with both doctors and outpatient nurses.

Designing the procedure

Many different hospital departments are usually involved in conducting and processing the results of investigations, including histopathology, haematology, cytology and radiology, and a result from any one of these departments could be the trigger for a patient to receive the cancer diagnosis. The research team had thought that it might be possible to use the histopathology department to advise them of impending bad news interviews, so that audit material could be put into the notes. A trial run was undertaken, and showed that this was not feasible for a number of reasons, including:

- histopathology was not the only department giving the critical result
- some cancers were diagnosed through specialist departments in other hospitals
- arrival of results on the ward was unpredictable
- some results were given by telephone.

Discussion with both ward and outpatient staff had shown that the situation on the wards was complex and unpredictable, with results arriving at irregular intervals, and no uniformity about what happens once they have arrived. The situation in outpatients is comparatively structured and predictable, and so it was decided that the guidelines would initially be tested out there. Clinic nurses are the key people in outpatients, and as they know in advance which patient are to receive bad news, the team decided to ask them to ensure that audit forms and other documentation were in the notes.

Designing the patient leaflet

One of the suggestions made by the working group was that patients should be given a personalised leaflet on which would be written the diagnosis, details of any tests to be undertaken, and a contact name and number for questions or problems. The researchers designed this leaflet [24] in collaboration with a patients representative; it was then sent to the local patient groups for comment.

Discussion

An overview of the second stage of the study is given below, including the drawing up of the guidelines and the designing of the audit process and interventions.

Establishing the guidelines

Taken as a whole, the process of establishing the guidelines can be seen as a successful one. A problem had been identified by means of consultation with patients, and the solution reached by the working group was agreeable to both patients and health professionals. The guidelines themselves are simple, require no special skills to implement, and are easily auditable. They are of course, only a partial solution to the problem of poor communication, but their use to identify those who could most benefit from additional training has potential within the field of postgraduate medical education and quality assurance.

The research team was fortunate to work in an area of medicine in which self-help groups are reasonably common. It was also able to build on earlier work done with the groups in the local area,[3] so that opinion could be easily consulted, and patient representatives could be identified who could draw on experiences other than their own for the purposes of the working group. Despite the comparative ease with which patients' views were obtained, a number of difficulties were encountered in carrying out the project.

As has been mentioned above, it is logistically difficult and time-consuming to arrange interviews with a large number of consultants. In addition, the range of experience and opinion is very great, and there were widely differing views on almost every topic discussed. In narrowing these views down so that they would be manageable by the working group, many subtleties were lost, and the resulting guidelines could be seen by some as over-simplified.

Logistical problems were also encountered in setting up the working group; finding mutually acceptable meeting times was always difficult, and the loss of two of the patient representatives meant that there was a danger that the professional view would take precedence.

The group was professionally facilitated, and the need for this became evident very early. The patient representatives found it difficult to penetrate the comfortable camaraderie of the professionals, and to comment on current practice without seeming over-critical or strident. The facilitator regularly had to intervene to enable them to overcome their diffidence.

Converting the results of the working group into auditable guidelines

The assistance of the clinical audit departments in this part of the study was invaluable. They were able to advise both on the feasibility of measuring certain activities, and on the wording of questions for the audit tools. In addition, because the personnel involved had experience of working as health professionals, they were able to clarify procedures and systems. The work done earlier in the study on the channels of communication and hospital systems enabled the team to assess the practicability of different options for auditing the implementation.

Designing the interventions

The standards established by the joint working group included the use of two new pieces of documentation, the referral proforma and the patient information leaflet. A draft referral proforma had already been designed by the breast surgery team at Hillingdon Hospital, and it included the medical information needed by the consultant, and some information for patients about what to expect when they attended the clinic for the first time. This leaflet is being revised to include information about the new patient-centred care Unit. No further work has been done on this intervention, partly for this reason, and partly because the research team had no knowledge or expertise in the field of general practice, and there was insufficient time for this to be researched. The team is nevertheless convinced of the potential value of such a proforma.

The patient information leaflet was successfully produced in collaboration with patients, and was used by the urology team as part of its piloting of the guidelines. Those patients who have been interviewed as part of the evaluation (see below) and who were given their diagnoses before this pilot, were asked whether they thought the leaflet would have been useful, and have all responded positively.

Chapter 4

Stage 3: Piloting and auditing the guidelines

Persuading clinicians to use the guidelines was the next stage of the project, and one for which major difficulties were anticipated. The researchers decided that the approach should be twofold:

- hospital managers would be asked about the possibility of the guidelines being adopted as trust-wide standards
- individual consultants who had been identified as both interested and influential would be asked to pilot the guidelines and interventions.

Working with hospital management

At the time of the project the two trusts involved (Mount Vernon and Watford Hospitals and the Hillingdon Hospital) were undertaking a number of organisational initiatives. Mount Vernon and Watford had recently merged and were also involved in a King's Fund Organisational Audit. At the same time The Hillingdon Hospital was implementing patient-centred care in its Women's Services division; this involved totally restructuring both outpatient and inpatient services, and included a major rebuilding programme in order to have all the relevant services available within a discrete area of the hospital. In view of this, it was necessary to adopt different means of implementing the guidelines.

Mount Vernon and Watford Hospitals NHS Trust

A quality team had recently been set up here, which comprised the executive board, the quality manager, representatives of purchasers and GPs, and consultants from the two hospitals. The researchers presented their work, and asked for advice on how to take it forward. The project was well received, and some consultants showed interest in the idea of a proforma for the referral of patients in whom cancer is suspected. No specific suggestions for the future were made, but the chief executive asked the researchers to give the quality team another presentation six months later, outlining progress.

The next initiative involved using the Organisational Audit as a background for implementation. It was noted that the use of the guidelines would fulfil a number of the criteria necessary for the accreditation of the Trust.

A letter has now been written by the project team to both the clinical and divisional directors for surgery, plastic surgery and medicine asking for the guidelines to be adopted throughout their respective divisions.

The Hillingdon Hospital

Two of the consultants who were involved in the doctor/patient working group are based at Hillingdon, and both work in women's services. For this reason, and also in order to test out the possibility of incorporating the guidelines into the Integrated Care Pathways (ICPs) which are an essential element in patient-centred care, the researchers decided to contact the patient-centred care co-ordinator.

A basic choice had to be made as to whether a separate communication ICP should be created, or whether existing ICPs should be adapted to take the guidelines into account. After discussion with a patient, it was agreed that the latter course should be adopted in order to prevent the 'communication' sheet from being ignored and also to give communication equal status with investigations and procedures.

The next step was to see whether it would be possible to adapt the existing ICPs which were in use for patients having investigations and/or surgery. Outpatient and inpatient breast patients were chosen, as the tests and surgical procedures are comparatively predictable.

Delays in the construction work and hence to the opening date of the patient-centred care unit from January 1995 to its eventual inauguration in July meant that no further progress was made in the adoption of the amended ICPs until October 1995. The divisional director for Women's Services has now agreed that, in collaboration with the acting manager of patient-centred care, the guidelines and personalised leaflet will be adapted to make them applicable to all new gynaecological diagnoses.

Working with individual consultants

Mount Vernon and Watford Hospitals NHS Trust

The researchers were advised by the clinical audit department that chances of success depended on working with a small number of consultants who were both interested in this approach and influential.

The consultants

The consultants asked to pilot the guidelines included: a physician/geriatrician, lead clinician for clinical audit; a plastic surgeon; a gastroenterologist; and general surgeon with special interest in the gastro-intestinal tract.

Each was asked to use the guidelines in his outpatient clinics, initially for a month, and to give each new cancer patient copies of the personalised leaflet, the Cancer Relief Macmillan Fund leaflet, *Help Is There*;[23] and *Coping with Your Cancer*.[23]

In addition they were asked to audit the communication process by completing one side of the audit form (see Appendix 4). The arrangement was confirmed by letter.

Once the consultants had agreed to take part, it was necessary to discuss the details of the arrangements with outpatient staff. The sisters in charge of each department were consulted, and they agreed that the clinic nurses would identify in advance the patients with a new cancer diagnosis, put copies of the relevant documentation into their notes, and complete and return the second side of the audit form. This discussion was again followed up by a letter confirming the details; a résumé of the procedure (see Appendix 5) was enclosed.

The Hillingdon Hospital

The medical teams who agreed to take part in the piloting of the guidelines at Hillingdon were the breast care team; the urology team; and gastroenterologist (the same consultant as in the Mount Vernon pilot).

Of these teams, only the breast care team is involved in the reorganisation leading to patient centred care; the other two were asked to take part because the urologists had already expressed an interest in the communication of bad news, and the gastroenterologist had been recruited through his work at Mount Vernon.

A process of consultation with key staff was undertaken here similar to that at Mount Vernon, with the oncologist acting as liaison between the research team and her medical colleagues.

Breast care team

This team has a breast surgeon and an associate specialist who has had both experience and specific training in the management of breast cancer. They work in close collaboration with a breast care nurse, who sees all newly diagnosed patients, and with a clinical oncologist. Part of the work of the team has recently been incorporated into the patient-centred care unit.

Urology team

A consultant and locum consultant, together with a nurse specialist all work closely with the clinical oncologist. The nurse specialist in this team had for some time been interested in improving the amount of support and information to men with bladder and prostate cancer, and was very keen to become involved in the study.

Problems encountered with the piloting and auditing process

Despite the care which had gone into planning how the guidelines would be piloted and audited, the process was fraught with complications. These were individually of a minor nature, but together they proved a major obstacle to achieving a satisfactory audit of the implementation of the guidelines in those clinics.

The problems encountered included the following:

- consultant unexpectedly on holiday
- clinic nurse on a day off and no-one else asked to implement procedure
- clinic floor being relaid
- teething problems with reorganisation of clinics
- clinic too busy for consultant to be reminded of procedure

- no new cancer patients in two out of four breast clinics
- uncertainty about changes in consultants' contracts
- lack of communication between consultants and their secretaries
- lack of communication between the two part-time secretaries to a consultant
- clinics cancelled at very short notice.

Although those who would be involved in the audit had been visited and had agreed that the procedure was helpful and manageable, these organisational problems have meant that of the clinics which originally agreed both the procedure and the timetable, only the urology clinic has regularly returned copies of the audit form; the only other clinic to send any forms back was the plastic surgery outpatient clinic, which sent two in two months.

Evaluating the guidelines and interventions

In order to evaluate the patients' perceptions of the guidelines and interventions, it was decided to interview a number of patients who had been told they had cancer two months earlier, and then to interview a similar number of those diagnosed following the introduction of the guidelines. The consultants were therefore asked to supply a list of patients from whom a small number could be selected for interview about the way they were told they had cancer. The response from the urology team was again prompt and efficient, with a full list of patients' names and addresses. A list was also received from the gastroenterologist at the Hillingdon. The patients on these lists were sent letters inviting them to participate in the interviews. At the time of writing, five patients had been interviewed. When asked their opinion of the personalised leaflet, all said that they would have found it helpful at the time of diagnosis.

A sample of patients who were diagnosed during the audit will be contacted two months after their diagnosis and interviewed about their experience of the bad news consultation. The intention is to compare these interviews with those of patients diagnosed before the introduction of the guidelines and personalised leaflet.

Discussion

The problems encountered can be attributable in large part to the context of the study. Major restructuring was under way in all three hospitals, and staff were involved in frequent and often disruptive changes. This frequently lead to problems with internal communication, and to a disinclination to become involved in yet another change in working practice. However, the NHS exists in an apparently permanent state of flux, and so it is essential that ways be found to motivate at least one senior member of the teams to take an active role in implementing such changes. The success of the urology team can be attributed to two factors:

- it is a small team, all of whom are committed to excellence in communication
- the support nurse, who is present at every clinic, takes responsibility for the 'small print' of audit, such as ensuring that the necessary paperwork is always available, and that the forms are filled in

● the team was set up from scratch, and working practices were designed collaboratively.

This team is an example of the 'sub-specialty team' envisaged by the Calman report.[1] In the future, cancer services in district general hospitals are likely to be organised in smaller specialist teams of this type; this reorganisation should create an infrastructure in which guidelines will become part of routine practice.

Chapter 5

Implications of the research findings

Training

The interviews with consultants demonstrated that there was considerable reluctance to undertake training in communication skills, even if it was designed specifically for consultants, and that many believed either that such skills cannot be taught or that they can be taught only on the job.

- Training in how to train junior staff was proposed as a way of both ensuring that consultants were familiar with the principles of good communication, and that they passed these on to their junior staff within everyday practice.
- The involvement of patients in the training of doctors was suggested as a way of ensuring that the patient's point of view was always addressed.

The following suggestions were made for increasing the participation of junior medical staff in communication skills training:

- consultants should insist on attendance
- work should be covered by other medical staff
- training should not be part of an already crammed induction course
- attendance should be a requirement without which accreditation would not be given.

The personalised leaflet

Although the patients interviewed generally felt that it would be helpful to have something in writing after their bad news interview, there was much less agreement among the consultants. The problem for most of the doctors lay less with the principle of giving written information than with the detail of what that information should be. Many were reluctant to give information about specific cancers, because such information would include details which could, at the stage of the initial diagnosis, be either irrelevant or overwhelming. They were, however, less anxious about letting patients know about sources of further information, as this would enable them to seek it at their own pace. The personalised leaflet was therefore designed to take account of these reservations.

The leaflet was designed specifically for use in outpatient departments, and has only been given out in only limited circumstances. However, the principle of giving patients written confirmation of what they have been told is applicable to any interview in which important information is given. Medical opinion is divided about how much to tell patients in the early stages of a disease; and the leaflet is therefore phrased 'the results of your tests show ...', so that the doctor has scope for clinical judgement.

Some of the information (e.g. details of the doctor's name and position, and the name and phone number of the person to contact for further information) is already applicable both to other medical conditions and to other settings. More specific information can be tailored to particular circumstances.

A number of amendments have been suggested, including:

- space for questions which the patient wishes to ask at the next consultation
- space for the patient to note symptoms or changes in his/her condition
- additional pages for subsequent consultations.

The team will be working with one of the doctors on the working group to make modifications to the leaflet.

Involving patients as volunteers in hospital

A number of patients commented favourably on the support they had gained from meeting other patients who had cancer, as they felt that someone who had been through the experience could offer them a unique insight, and that they were encouraged by meeting a cancer patient who was still alive.

The involvement of support group members in outpatient clinics and on the wards is very much in its infancy. It is regarded with suspicion by many professionals, who see the volunteer as a well-meaning amateur, or perceive support group members as a threat. However, the experience of this project indicates that suitably trained volunteers would have a great deal to contribute to the emotional and practical support of newly diagnosed cancer patients, and ways should be sought of making use of their expertise.

The guidelines as a model for other bad news interviews

In their present form, the guidelines are only intended for use when the first diagnosis of cancer is given. As was pointed out very forcefully by a number of consultants, however, this is far from being the only occasion on which patients are given bad news, and the underlying principles remain the same in any situation of this type. Apart from the specific reference to using the word 'cancer' and avoiding euphemisms, the guidelines in their present form could, in fact, be applied on any occasion when patients are given a potentially distressing diagnosis, and they could easily be adapted to be more specific to a particular condition.

One consultant pointed out that they represent 'only common sense and courtesy', but it seems that even these two attributes are not always in evidence when patients are told things which are potentially distressing. Communicating complex and possibly traumatic information to patients needs considerable skill. However, giving information of this type often has to be done by people who have neither the personality to do it naturally nor the inclination to learn to improve. In these circumstances the most that can be hoped for is that they avoid the major pitfalls. Common sense and courtesy combined with some planning of the interview should be enough to ensure that no disasters occur, and the guidelines are designed to ensure that such basic standards are maintained.

The project as a model for patient involvement

There are many areas of health service provision in which both professionals and patients are able to identify shortcomings, but where mutually agreeable solutions have proved elusive. If changes are to be implemented, they must take into account the views and experiences both of the consumers and the providers of services. Historically, changes in service provision have resulted from decisions made by professionals about what they consider to be the needs of patients. The trend is now in the direction of greater user involvement, but this is not always easy to achieve.

The methods used in this project, although time-consuming, have proved successful in incorporating the views of both users and providers in finding mutually acceptable solutions. The model can be summarised as follows.

- Identification and involvement of key staff.
- Feedback from patients using qualitative techniques.
- Feedback from professionals using qualitative techniques.
- Facilitated, task-oriented joint working group.

If relationships exist with local patient groups, then the patient feedback will be quicker and easier to obtain, as will patient representatives who are used to drawing on experiences other than their own. Such relationships should therefore be nurtured whenever possible.

Chapter 6

Conclusions

The work has generated a considerable amount of interest both among those who have taken part and among colleagues. The delays and frustrations described in the report have meant that the impact of the work is only now beginning to be seen within the three hospitals involved, but the team are confident that, at least at Hillingdon, a major breakthrough has been made. Divisional directors at Mount Vernon and Watford Hospitals NHS Trust have also responded favourably to the ideas contained in the guidelines.

The study was presented by Dr Jane Maher, project director, at the joint annual conference of the British Oncological Association and the British Association for Surgical Oncology. The session was very well attended, and large numbers of the printed guidelines were taken away by delegates. A paper is in preparation outlining the model developed for involving patients and professionals in producing guidelines.

Many of the difficulties experienced by both patients and doctors in the breaking of bad news can be overcome by the use of basic guidelines for the organisation and planning of the interview. Problems of communication are not necessarily too complex to be addressed in this way, and the solutions suggested are measurable can be used by practitioners without specialist training.

Patients and professionals can work fruitfully together to find mutually acceptable solutions to a problem, but this needs careful planning and facilitation. The developing and nurturing of relationships with patient groups are crucial to their future involvement.

The implementation of such solutions may presents organisational problems which involve all the members of a medical team. Such problems may well appear trivial, but the implementation of change requires close attention to even the smallest of details.

The reorganisation of cancer services in district general hospitals in the wake of the Calman report will result in the creation of small sub-specialty teams. These offer an opportunity for the adoption of guidelines for the communication of the cancer diagnosis, as well as for the development of agreed protocols for referral and treatment. Patient involvement at this level has yet to be tried, but would mean that services could be organised in a way which truly reflects the wishes of users.

References

1. *A policy framework for commissioning cancer services.* Department of Health, 1995

2. Bradburn J, Maher EJ, Young J, Young T. Community based cancer support groups: an undervalued resource. *Clinical Oncology* 1992; 4:377–80

3. Bradburn J. Linking hospital and community support groups. *Journal of Cancer Care* 1992; 1:179–81

4. Maguire P. Can communication skills be taught? *Br J Hospital Medicine* 1990; 43:215–16

5. *Consumer Audit Guidelines.* College of Health, 1994

6. *What seems to be the matter: communication between hospitals and patients.* Audit Commission, 1993

7. Bradburn J, Maher EJ. The growth of advocacy groups for cancer patients in Europe and America. *Oncology Today* 1995; 12:14–17

8. Frederickson L, Bull P. An appraisal of the current status of communication skills in British Medical Schools. *Social Science & Medicine* 1992; 34:515–22

9. Finlay I, Dallimore D. Your child is dead. *BMJ* 1991; 302:1524–5

10. Seale C. Communication & awareness about death; a study of a random sample of dying people. *Social Science & Medicine* 1991; 32:943–52

11. Rethans J-J, Drop R, Sturmans F, van der Leuten C. Assessment of the performance of general practitioners by the use of standardised (simulated) patients. *British Journal of General Practice* 1991; 41:97–9

12. Hays RB. Assessment of general practice consultations: content validity of a rating scale. *Medical Education* 1990; 24:110–16

13. Cox J, Mulholland H. An instrument for assessment of videotapes of general practitioners' performance. *BMJ* 1993; 306:1043–6

14 Maguire P, Fairbairn S, Fletcher C. Communication skills of young doctors I. *BMJ* 1986; 292:153–6

15 Maher EJ, Jefferis AF. Decision making in advanced cancer of the head & neck: variation in the views of medical specialists. *Journal of the Royal Society of Medicine*, June 1990

16 Maguire P. Barriers to psychological care of the dying. *BMJ* 1985; 291:1711–13

17 Wilkinson S. Factors which influence how nurses communicate with cancer patients. *Journal of Advanced Nursing* 1991; 16:677–88

18 Maguire P, Fairbairn S, Fletcher C. Communication skills of young doctors II. *BMJ* 1986; 292: 1576–8

19. Hogbin B, Fallowfield L. Getting it taped: the 'bad news' consultation with cancer patients. *British Journal of Hospital Medicine* 1989; 41:330–3

20. Lewis SW, McHugh P, Fallowfield L, Ford S. Do audiotapes help cancer patients? A randomised, controlled trial. BPOG Annual conference Guy's Hospital, 1993

21 Woolley H, Stein A, Forrest GC, Baum JD. Imparting the diagnosis of life threatening illness in children. *BMJ* 1989; 298:1623–6

22. Mount Venon Centre for Cancer Treatment. *Coping with Your Cancer. A self-help guide.* Mount Vernon & Watford Hospitals NHS Trust, 1995.

23. Cancer Relief Macmillan Fund. *Help Is There. National contacts for people with cancer.* Cancer Relief Macmillan Fund, 1995.

24. Patient Involvement Unit, Lynda Jackson Macmillan Centre for Cancer Support and Information, Mount Vernon Hospital. *Patient Information Card.* King's Fund, 1996.

Appendix 1

Quotations from patients

Preparation for the diagnosis

This young woman, who was 31 years old when diagnosed with breast cancer, had had an aspiration which indicated that her breast lump was benign. As a result, both she and her doctor were fairly confident that the removal of the lump was routine. However it was found to be cancerous. She said she was 'very shaken, particularly as it seemed as if it was going to be routine. I did feel then that I was too young for something like this to happen. I've always been healthy. I had no reason to believe I'd have a problem like this ... it was just a terrible shock.'

'Obviously you talk to people about it and to your nearest relatives. Everybody said it'll just be a little cyst, lots of women have these and I got it firmly implanted in my mind, just a little cyst that would be taken away and there would be no more trouble, so that when I was told, it was quite a shock ...'

'I had mastitis and kept going back to my GP and eventually he thought he could feel something sinister ... he was 99 per cent certain it was a cyst.'

'He [the surgeon] said, well I must have been a bit thick or something, he said, "It looks very suspicious ..." I didn't click that he meant it was really suspicious, I thought when it's been tested he'll find it's not. I got it in my mind that it wasn't going to be anything like that.'

'When I had a bronchoscopy, I said to the registrar, "What's down there?" She said, "As soon as we have it [the results], we'll tell you." So afterwards, I was sitting there absolutely knackered and I said, "Well, what's down there?" "Oh I can't tell you now." And I said, "Well you told me you were going to." And she said, "Oh no, it's got to be sent off for biopsies. All I am willing to say to you is that there is a hell of a lot of activity down there." Well that said it all, really. But I was still keeping an open mind – I didn't want to hear it, I didn't even want to think about it. All I kept saying was, "No, I'm going to be all right, it's an infection, it's an abscess because that's what they were testing for." But I think you do know really, you just don't want to admit it to yourself.'

'There was no time to worry about it. I was told all in one go. There was no "do one thing one minute and then come back in two weeks' time" – you don't live in that time – you just exist. I was lucky I didn't know anything beforehand. I didn't have the anxiety. You don't want to wait to know.'

'I knew exactly what it was. I was outside thinking, "I'm almost certain it is but perhaps it isn't, hopefully." I think that it helped a lot, knowing or thinking this definitely is cancer. It wasn't such a blow. But to somebody who thought it was just lumpiness, it might have been.'

'He was a very good specialist and he did prepare us for the worst. There were lots of tears that week, "Why me?" – you know, and then this morning I saw Dr ... and it all came out again, more tears ... I thought, "I'm prepared for the worst", but it's all confirmed ... it wasn't that bad experience, in a sense, being told, really ... I don't know how it could have been told really. He didn't beat about the bush. He said, "You're having a really bad day, aren't you?" I don't know if it could be done better. My partner held my hand.'

'It is important that people are aware of what it might be before the biopsy.'

'Perhaps when the surgeon comes round after the operation he should say, "We're going to test the tumour and you should be aware that it might be malignant". I don't like being kept in the dark; it's my body and it's therefore important that I know these things'.

Doctor's manner/attitude

'I've got cancer – if doctors are dealing with adults they should treat them like adults and if they have something to say they should say it. There is nothing to be gained by wrapping things up in a parcel.'

'I turned my head the other way and he did the biopsy and told me to get dressed ... He sat himself behind his desk with his little bottle in front of him ... He never said, "Have you got someone with you, do you want to bring your husband in?" ... not a thing. He just looked at the bottle and said, "Well, from my experience, looking at the way it's reacting I would say that it's definitely malignant and there's only one thing – that's a total mastectomy." And that was it.'

'He didn't know me from Adam, he didn't know whether he was going to end up with a gibbering female on his hands going to pieces and I suppose in one respect, if you do it like this she hasn't got time to collapse and have the screaming habdabs or anything ... But it's still an awful shock to the system to be told so bluntly ... there were no preliminaries, or "Maybe we could do this" and "If it's that, maybe we could do something else".'

'"I'm this and I'm that, I'm the specialist and I'll tell you what's happening." I was not keen to see him because I shall be all tensed up and I don't really want that. I don't want to get tensed up for anybody or anything. Why should I get tensed up over a doctor?'

'You can ask him anything and he'll tell you and nothing's too much trouble ... And he's light with it ... There again if you want to talk in depth with him, he'll talk in depth ... He's friendly with it, I don't know how to put it into words, but I think he's user friendly.'

'My overriding feeling towards him is respect and affection ... he had this very caring and concerned attitude and I feel he really does care what is going on with me.'

'Everything you asked you got a straight answer and you were treated as if you had a bit of common sense, a bit of intelligence. Also, she fitted us in at the end of a very busy clinic and saw us at half past eight at night. As we walked in she said, "I'm sorry to keep you waiting" and she said, "Now you're here there's no hurry, take your time, ask any questions you want".'

Doctor did not know me/lack of rapport

'I had never seen this doctor before. I was in Northwick Park and this consultant who had been brought from Mount Vernon to Northwick Park ... he was a complete stranger. People want to be told on their own terms ... that's why I think the relationship with the doctor or carer needs to be established.'

'I was just fortunate I suppose. He was an elderly gentleman with a lovely bedside manner. He was very quiet, but he answered my questions. Now he gives me a hug and a kiss. You get to know them as you go along. It's a totally different relationship a year on than it is that first day.'

'But the surgeon who told me – he was excellent really because he wasn't ...he was very down to earth. He didn't say, "I'm terribly sorry." He just said, "Well I'm afraid it's cancer".'

'I mean you don't know the people you're dealing, with so that makes it difficult because if you know the sort of person you've got ... it's like with the children I have at school. If you know the sort of child he is then you know how to approach him and how to say things.'

'It must be very difficult for the person in that position who doesn't really know the person they're talking to and how they are going to react. His way is probably the best way – very down to earth and "I'm sorry but I'm afraid it is cancer,"- adding straightaway, "but I can see you're shocked but there's lots we can do about it".'

'If you go to your own doctor you know him, he knows you, you get a better rapport'.

Language

'His [the doctor's] words were, "Prepare yourself for the worst, I think it's a tumour." So he didn't actually come out with the word "cancer" and it was only when I went to see my mum that I said, "Does that mean it's cancer?".'

'Cancer wasn't mentioned till Mr ... said, "It's a growth, it's cancer." I feel now that people have got to accept the word "cancer" – it's fear of the unknown.'

'In my opinion doctors are oversensitive, they're frightened of the word "cancer".'

'I had a friend who was told it was a carcinoma, now she made the link that meant cancer, but why didn't they say cancer? It's like giving it a special power if you don't say the horrible word.'

'I couldn't bear the word "cancer" so I couldn't bear to read anything about it or watch the television, but as time goes by you can. Now I can read anything, I just think, "I'm an individual" and let them treat me as an individual and I can't really compare myself with other people.'

'I remember most that it was not explained properly – just, "You've got pleomorphic adenoma." They said it was not malignant but might become malignant ... I don't think it was explained properly.' This patient asked for the word to be written down, and went and looked it up in the library. 'It was quite straightforward what the words meant, they should have been able to explain the words, they were just dressing it up in medical gobbledy gook.'

Having someone with you

'I've done it mostly on my own. I don't know whether that's because I thought he [her husband] would be upset or I felt I could cope with it on my own.'

'My husband was having a lot of business troubles when my diagnosis was made and I've always said that he can do enough worrying for the two of us, so I didn't want to concern him with anything.'

'I would have needed somebody there. You just become a zombie. You have all these emotions, about treatment – "It'll hurt, I'll die." He [the doctor] said he'd discuss the treatment but I couldn't really take it in. Coming home I was in a dream. I wouldn't have been able to drive home.'

'The difference is, if somebody's telling you about it [the diagnosis] you're not really listening, you don't know. You don't know what questions to ask anyway. If someone else is there they listen, hear what was said and ask the right questions.'

'I came out and told my daughter and got reassured straightaway. I thought, well I've got the kids to worry about. If I'd been on my own I think I might have gone into a state or something. I might have cried all the way home on the bus or something but she had the car. I was so glad that she was there because when you hear that you've got this non-Hodgkins lymphoma, you think, "Well what on earth is that", but she was so calm. They reassured me. In the end we had a laugh about it, but if I'd been on my own I wouldn't have asked. I was so glad she came, if my husband had come, he wouldn't have asked questions. It was so reassuring, she said, "Mum, you've just got to carry on as normal".'

'All the way through I was told it wasn't going to be malignant, that it was just a benign lump ... A friend offered to come with me and I thought, "No" because I shall feel so stupid. So I didn't take her up on her offer. My husband never thinks there's anything wrong unless it's happened, so I went along on my own. It's like a lottery. If we knew before we went that we were going to be told we had cancer, then we could decide if we wanted somebody there or not! But ... it's a matter of chance whether you've got what you want – someone with you or on your own.'

The needs of relatives

'I think it might lead to problems between the partners of people with cancer because there's a barrier there, isn't there; there's something between you, a terrible secret that's not being discussed and it must affect the way that you are with each other. It must be a terrible strain to keep something like that from somebody.'

'My husband [the patient] was the one who said we should have been told together – we're grown up people, we're not children.'

'I think if it's bad news – the partner or close relative, a close friend if the person hasn't got anybody – they should be brought together and it should be a peaceful atmosphere and it should be given in a nice way and there should be someone there you can talk to. I don't expect it to be with specialists because they're busy ... but somebody there that they can talk to, a counsellor or a nurse or somebody who could then take the time to be with you, just to get over the shock and perhaps enable you to ask questions, or at least someone you could go back to later ... but you're just left, just chopped off. You don't know what to do.'

Support

'[You need] an angel on hand, who will take you and give you a cup of tea, time to collect yourself – I came out of hospital and I felt demented. You feel like a bat out of hell, I couldn't even think of a taxi number – if there was transport, it would help.'

This woman who had been unaccompanied explained that there was no specialist nurse in post at the hospital at the time (a year ago) and that she was sent off round the hospital for tests in a daze. A nurse had taken her to the admissions office, but left her to find pharmacy and have a chest X-ray because she had to get back to another patient. She was given no leaflets. She said, 'All I had were X-ray forms, blood test forms.' She had not been asked how she was getting home – 'I don't remember the journey home. I drove myself home and I don't remember the journey. It's horrific when I look back and I think what I could have done. I could have so easily caused an accident ... I wasn't behaving very sensibly because I've got friends on the end of the phone and I could have phoned them to take me home ... but then I wasn't in a logical mood. I was definitely in shock so I just did everything automatically – I'd got to get to these departments and I'd got to get home.'

'What was particularly useful was that she saw me at that initial stage and she was here [later, at the patient's home] three hours and talked through all the treatment options and well, just the emotional worries – I mean I was particularly worried. I've got three young children and I've got a daughter who's disabled, and I was very worried about her because immediately you conclude you're going to die. But having talked to her and talked to the consultant and realised that that's not necessarily the case and I was lucky it was detected early and that you've got to start thinking more positively. When you're into the process of discussing it and treatment then you calm down about it, but that initial shock – I felt that I needed to discuss it in detail straight away. I couldn't wait because there were so many questions racing around in my brain. I wanted those questions answered more or less straight away because I didn't know anything about cancer before that and the Macmillan nurse in particular was just brilliant. Such a big support. I feel as if she really helped me in those early stages.'

'I didn't think the Macmillan nurse was very good, she said, "Have a cup of tea, you'll be all right, don't you worry about it," and she stayed a little while and then off she went. Oh! and she gave us a card and said, "Phone me anytime I'm here, or phone me at home".'

'I found I lacked that. I had my Mum if I was down and I phoned BACUP and they found someone who'd had the same as me and that was a great help – feeling that the feelings I had were normal, and I got information.'

'I remember going in for a lumpectomy and the breast care nurse came to talk to me at my bedside. I can't remember now what she spoke to me about – I think I was too nervous – but I felt at the time that I couldn't relate to her, she was too young. But I got to know Mary [fellow group member] and I think she's the one who helped me most because she's been through the experience herself and talked to me a lot and gave me booklets.'

'I've had no consultation at all from my GP, nothing. I went for the initial one with the lump, she sent me to hospital. She never phoned, no-one phoned from the surgery and it's only recently that I've been back to her. She tells me that they've had good results from the hospital about me, but they [the GPs] don't come, you don't get anything from them afterwards.'

'You go to your GP and that's it, they're finished with it; you go to the surgeon, that's it, that's finished with; you go to have radiotherapy, that's someone else again ... I have seen the oncologist ever since at regular intervals. So he's the only continuity I've had. But everywhere else it's not followed through at all is it? ... Going back to your GP ... you should go and make an appointment and go and sit and discuss it with him, or even the practice nurse or something. But when you're totally green, you don't know anything about anything, you just need information, you're starved of information.'

Other things happening in people's lives

'My mother was 92 , and was ill for four months before she died and I was racing up and down to hospital. Then the dog was put to sleep ... It was just a nightmare'. [Her mother died before treatment started.] 'She did me a good turn really because I didn't know how I was going to get to Mount Vernon every day and then back again to see my mother'. [Her surgeon was unaware of these difficulties.] 'Well I mean, I didn't say, well you don't really go into all that do you?'

Information, treatment and choice

'He [the doctor] mentioned to me the word "cancer" and my mind went blank.'

'Maybe he did explain things, but I didn't hear.'

'You go a bit blank. You don't take everything in and I think you should have some lifeline there. There should be some information that gives somewhere you can phone, write ... so that you can say, "Help! What's happening?".'

'Once you talk to someone you're focused on a plan of action and so you're moving forward, you're in this sort of no man's land until you talk to someone like that. You feel as if someone's put this sort of death sentence on you and you just don't know how to come to terms with it, but it seems everything's in a fog. Your thoughts are not clear at all, and once I'd talked to someone in detail about it I felt as if I could clarify what was going to happen, what the future was going to hold,the problem was going to be resolved. I was extremely frightened about having chemotherapy; it's silly really but the only thing I could relate it to was that awful film about Bob Champion the jockey ... those awful pictures came up in my mind; but once I'd talked to someone in detail about it, that put that into perspective, and it took away the fear . You realize that it's not like that anymore. People don't even always lose their hair and that there are drugs to control sickness. Talking it over helps to control the fear I suppose'.

'Nobody explains why you have it all – why have I had radiotherapy, chemotherapy?'

'The biggest problem is, for a lot of people, on their first visit to the hospital they are not streetwise, or however you like to define it ... He [the doctor] didn't say he was from Mount Vernon, which he was, and so I got quite a shock on the Wednesday when I got a call at work to say "Can you be in at Mount Vernon at eleven o'clock tomorrow morning, and we will operate Friday." I'd been thinking that I was going to Northwick Park, so nothing was explained to me at all ... he told me his name but I didn't know I was seeing a surgeon.'

'I didn't know they'd removed my lymph glands until a long, long while afterwards. And I didn't even know I'd had what they call a radical mastectomy. I just thought I'd had a mastectomy. I didn't even know that there were different types of mastectomy.'

A positive message

'His way is probably the best way – very down to earth and "I'm sorry but I'm afraid it is cancer," but straightaway "but I can see you're shocked but there's lots we can do about it." And then he was very up, up, then and he said, "Well, it's not the end, you have a choice whether you have the whole breast off or part of it off" and he gave me time to go away and think about it.'

'I think it would be a good idea, not just to turn round and say, "OK you've got cancer", but to say, "There's a lot being done with cancer over the last few years. It isn't like it used to be. We have treatments now. There are lots of different ways it can be dealt with." To give people hope so they don't go away and think, "I've got cancer, I'm going to die." They've got to think positive.'

Privacy and vulnerability

'I remember people taking sidelong glances.'

'The surgeon came round the ward and went to everybody in the ward and looked at their bed and said, "See you in the morning" to everyone, and he looked across at me and he said, "I'll come and have a talk with you later." I thought, "Why am I different?" It wasn't how he treated everybody else. When later he came, he walked up and it felt to me as though before he even spoke there was something different going on, different to everybody else – and of course it was, it was cancer. I felt that he was separating me from everybody else. I suppose he pulled the curtains round because he was wondering how I'd react – whether I'd be hysterical, or cry or upset the others, or he didn't want me to be seen upset by the others.' Afterwards she said she 'lay and thought about things, and then I got down under the bedclothes and I did have a cry because I realised what was happening. This nurse came up to me and said, "Are you all right? Would you like a cup of tea?" and I said I would, so I had a cup of tea.'

'I would not have made a fool of myself normally'. After the doctor had gone she said that she was 'very very tearful. A lady from across the way saw that I was upset and she came over and chatted to me for a minute. Then the nurse came and she drew the curtains round and gave me a cuddle. She could see I was in tears and she just said, "I think you need a cuddle" and she was a lovely nurse.'

'There's one thing I always find and that is, when you're very very low or not at all well, not able to think – that's when they tell you. You're not prepared, you don't know what to say or what to do.'

'There's nothing worse than being flat on your back with the consultant standing feet above, looking down at you, trying to say something important. Even sitting, and he's standing. You need to be eyeball to eyeball ... You feel more a human being where you're in a vertical position rather than a horizontal one.'

'I was sitting with the top half of me naked and he [the doctor] said it was a tumour and it was malignant. I felt very vulnerable. As he was just saying it the nurse who was sitting behind me, picked up my cardigan and put it round my shoulders which was a nice touch – I appreciated that very much.'

'I was shown into the examination room and they say, "Take off your top and get ready" and to oblige, you do. I spent twenty minutes to half an hour just lying there ... there you are, lying on your back with your breasts bare ... next minute you're out of the door.'

Time

'I don't think it's the time, I think it's what's said.'

Mrs B. said that her friend was asked to leave by the doctor as she wished to speak to the patient alone. 'I said 'If it's important, could you wait for my husband and son and daughter?' The consultant told her that a member of her own family was ill and that she therefore could not wait. She then told Mrs B. that she had a malignant cancer and said 'Well I must go now.' I thought 'This doctor's mad!' I got hot. I got this flush and I had my dressing gown on. I looked around, I thought the doctor was talking to someone else, so I said 'You're not talking to me, it can't be me!', and the doctor said 'Well it is'. I thought I was going crackers. Then the doctor left and left me with this young nurse. I said 'Will you stay with me until my husband and son and daughter come back?' They came in about 10 minutes time – the doctor could have waited until they came to break the news'. Mrs B finished by saying that she had never complained about the way she was told but was very upset about it.

When patients 'discover' their diagnosis

Mrs G had been referred with a breast lump to a consultant who had examined her and told her that he thought there would be no problem. She returned to see him in six weeks, the lump was a big bigger. He had done an aspiration and the results came back which indicated that it was benign, but he had advised her to have the lump removed, which it was. She said, 'It seemed as if it was going to be a routine thing, no problem.' She made a clinic appointment for a few weeks later when she would receive the biopsy results. 'Then a couple of days before that, I'd had a phone call from the clinic to say that the consultant, who was my consultant, could I go and see him the following day. So this was just the appointments clerk who phoned up and immediately my heart stopped because I knew there must be some problem because that would be the only reason they'd want me to go immediately for an appointment. I said was there any difficulty so she said, "No difficulty. Mr ... wants to see you tomorrow." I thought there's no point in asking her. My mind was immediately in a complete whizz. I put the phone down and I immediately thought I was going to collapse on the spot and my legs turned to jelly. I phoned to my husband at work and said this had happened and that I'd got cancer, and he said, "Well don't panic, I'm coming home, and I'll phone our doctor (which is our GP) and get him to phone the hospital and find out." Because I said I can't wait until tomorrow, I'll go mad not knowing. Fortunately my GP is very good. He did manage to get in touch with the hospital and he spoke to the hospital. He said, "Yes, it was a cancer," and he arranged to come round to the house and talk to us that evening, which he did and he was very good. He gave me a sleeping pill and then the following day I went to see the consultant. I don't think it's a good idea to be phoned up cold from the clinic like that. I don't know how practical it is to have a home visit, but I certainly found that very useful. I suppose it's easier to feel relaxed in your own home environment.'

Mrs L. who had ovarian cancer said that she had been to her GP 'who was trying to convince me I was pregnant for four or five weeks. Eventually I got past the GP and got this doctor who did an ultrasound and said, "There's something here, but I can't tell you what it is, we've got to open you up." She said that she felt there must be something wrong as she had not had any menstrual problems but was facing a hysterectomy. By the time she was ready for the operation she was huge. 'A nurse came up to me the night before the operation. I was walking around looking heavily pregnant wearing one of those kaftans and she said, "Don't think you're the only one with fibroids that size. I've seen bigger." and that momentarily gave me a lift – gosh she has seen bigger. It is a fibroid!' However, Mrs L. felt it could not be fibroids as she had had no menstrual problems leading up to it. 'Halfway through the week post-operatively, the penny dropped. I thought I was the only one who had to stay in for her results and nobody else had, and I thought, "This isn't right," and the penny dropped and it all made sense and I literally diagnosed myself. I got in a state and the sister came and pulled the curtains and said, "Well it's good for you to think like this," and I thought, "My God, that's it!" And that was it. Then on the seventh morning, the surgeon came and he actually told me. It was a very nice room attached to the ward and I knew he was coming and what he had to say. He's a brilliant surgeon, but not a very good bedside manner. So I actually helped him – even with the diagnosis – and it was fine. There was a sister and a nurse there, they were both looking at me and waiting for me to crack, to go through the ceiling. For some reason I was very calm and collected because I felt I'd been there, I'd had the initial shock brought on by myself.'

Quotations from doctors

Communication skills training

'I did my training before communication skills, computers or management skills.'

'W S (the consultant he had worked for) taught me everything I know. I don't do it the way he did but I use his techniques.'

'Medical school and seeing patients has been my training. You can't teach communication skills any more than you can teach management. You can either do it or you can't.'

'There's too much training for people, telling them how to do their job.'

'A bad cook who goes to cookery classes only becomes an educated bad cook.' This may still be an improvement, however.

'It's easy to say you're experienced but that doesn't necessarily mean you're very good at it.'

'In principle I'd come – if Dr X [another consultant] said he thought I needed it I would go. If management told me I'd give them two fingers. I'd probably go to sleep at the back.'

'It's very difficult to train consultants to do *anything* .'

Who gives the news

'We all take a share but I see the primary responsibility as mine.'

'There's the aspect of continuity for the patient and family. Junior doctors come and go but the consultant is always there.'

'If a consultant's response is 'I can't have you in the interview' it probably means he's nowhere near good enough to be doing it himself.'

Telling the news by telephone

'God I hope not. I can't think there's anyone I'd tell anything to over the phone.'

'Doctors often pressure you into giving news over the phone but I always refuse. That's a rule for me.'

'No – you can't be certain you're speaking to the patient.'

'It's not my practice but it does happen when patients put you under pressure.'

'It's inappropriate but it can be expedient.'

'Yes, I frequently do ... I'd only do it of course if I knew the patient well'.

The content of the interview

'You have to discuss the treatment options – it's like a psychiatrist, you can't take someone's personality to bits without being able to put it back together. So you can't tell someone something like that and destroy them without giving them something to hold on to.'

'The patients need to know that I understand. We've got to hold hands to the end.'

Process and preparation

'Telling isn't a single episode.'

'The Senior Registrar and Registrar dot the i's and cross the t's because the patients often don't take in everything that's said. Once the news is broken they don't hear the rest.'

'If the patient's having a biopsy then they know something's up.'

'Some people don't want to discuss their anxieties until the diagnosis is certain.'

'In a very busy clinic you often really don't know what to expect. X-ray reports come inside a packet and you open it all together when the patient is in the room. You don't have time to assess how the patient will take the news.'

The importance of the bad news interview

'It's unspeakably important – on a scale of 1 to 10 it's off the end. It's important as a humanitarian gesture and for creating trust and empathy for the future'.

'It's probably the most important clinical thing I do. It's got to set the framework for the treatment.'

'It's very fundamental really, because if it goes wrong it prejudices relationships with all the people who provide care.'

'It's not important or unimportant. It's something you have to do ... It's a matter of basic interview technique.'

What the consultants found difficult

'It's one of the hardest things you have to do because you're trained to be optimistic and positive.'

'It's always difficult because it is bad news.'

'It's no easier now than it was when I was first qualified.'

'It's something you don't actually find difficult to do because you are doing it all the time, but it's a difficult area for doctor/patient communication.'

Specific difficulties

'Occasionally they break down, and that's terrible.'

'People being horrible to me – that's the worst.. I know it's only grief making them angry, but it's very upsetting.'

'Please let your patient groups know that this is the most difficult thing of all. It becomes impossible for doctors and nurses, because you can't just say you're going to take a biopsy – you have to give a reason. You can put that in triplicate to your patient groups'.

Confidence

'How do you decide at the end of the day whether you've done it well?'

Time

'If there are forty patients waiting in the clinic you can't spend 20 minutes or more doing a bad news interview.'

'The clinic is always very rushed and hasty. It's designed for the surgeon's convenience and not for the comfort of the patient.'

'I make time. For a patient with cancer of the oesophagus it can take up to an hour. It's very complicated and there are many ways of treating it, and in the end it has to be the patient's choice. Time is a problem for the other patients in the clinic and for the nurses who run it.'

Lack of knowledge of the patient

'One of the major deficiencies in hospital is that you don' t know enough about the patient's background.'

'... not understanding enough of the person's inner attitude.'

Problems of comprehension

'You have to tell the patient, but of course nine out of ten don't understand a word you say.'

'They hear the news of cancer and then they don't hear anything else you say.'

Opinions about the use of guidelines in communication

'I object very strongly to guidelines. They stop people thinking. If you need guidelines you shouldn't be doing it.'

'Personally I'm not really a conformist. I lay down my own guidelines by taking junior staff along to see how I do it ... I just think that kind of thing is appalling. I can't stand rules being laid down in that area.'

'The bottom line is all about litigation – how your peers would have acted in the same situation. It's very important to write them to allow a reasonable spread of behaviour by clinicians.'

'We could and should write standards, and they should include support for the hearer and the giver.'

Guidelines

'If the patient's been alive for 50 years, they don't need to be told they're dying in a minute.'

'It's best if they're dressed, then they're not at your mercy. When someone's got no clothes on, they feel more vulnerable.'

'We often draw the curtains round and kid ourselves that there's privacy – but there's not really privacy, there's contact by sound and even sometimes by sight because the curtains are so far off the floor.'

'You mustn't promise the earth, but the patient needs some hope.'

'If you tell the truth then there aren't problems. If the patient denies it then there *are* problems. If the news isn't well received there's not much you can do about it.'

'If you're nice and kindly and say 'a few nasty cells' or 'a little shadow on the X-ray then the patients may well be none the wiser. But if you say, "Hello, well you've got cancer" then at least they know, although they may feel it's been done very insensitively.'

'Whatever you're doing you must be concentrating, you must give it your full attention.'

'You have to match the English to the individual, but sometimes you can go *through* words to understanding.'

Quotations from members of the working group

'People are unbelievably obsequious and afraid of questioning or asking in case they should feel silly or foolish if they ask this question. Just to tell people that it's OK , that the thing is for you to go out of the room feeling happy and with your questions answered in a way that's suitable to you, in language you understand, and if you don't understand to ask for an explanation ... We need to tell people that the time that they are in there is their time.'

Doctor: 'What is very salutary is to go to a support group and I'm not sure if all junior staff shouldn't do this. You certainly learn what it is that worries people.'
Patient: 'Why? Because we are no different from you.'
Doctor: 'Yes, but in the hospital we are different, aren't we? When we go into your territory, it's quite a different relationship. That's why it's so salutary.'
Counsellor: 'But then it's no different from when the patient comes into the hospital and is overawed by the doctors.'

'If I've got to see someone who has had a bad diagnosis broken to them it's really helpful to know what was said because although you can take it from where the patient is at that time it's very difficult to see what the gap is [in the patient's appreciation of the situation].'

Audit form

Name	No:
	Patient Label
Address	

Doctor/Patient Communication Audit

Nurse:

	Yes	No
Was the patient seen by a senior member of the medical team?	☐	☐
Did the doctor prepare in advance for the consultation by reading results?	☐	☐
Were arrangements made to minimise interruptions to the consultation?	☐	☐
Was the phone diverted?	☐	☐
Was the bleep/pager given to another member of the team?	☐	☐

Other, please give example...

....

	Yes	No
Was a support nurse involved?	☐	☐

If not, was it because:

	Yes	No
a) not in post	☐	☐
b) not available	☐	☐
c) not invited	☐	☐
d) other	☐	☐

	Yes	No
Did the patient bring a friend or relative to the clinic?	☐	☐
If not, was the patient asked about how they were getting home?	☐	☐

Doctor:

	Yes	No
Were all results available?	☐	☐

If no, which were unavailable? ....

....

	Yes	No
Did you make formal introductions?	☐	☐
Was the patient sitting up and dressed when you gave the bad news?	☐	☐

If no, why not? ....

....

	Yes	No
Did you ask the patient what he/she thought the problem might be?	☐	☐

When you gave the diagnosis did you use the word 'cancer'

	Yes	No
a) verbally?	☐	☐
b) in writing?	☐	☐

If not, why? ....

....

	Yes	No
Did you refer the patient to another specialist for treatment?	☐	☐
If no, did you discuss the treatment options you could offer?	☐	☐
Do you think the patient understood the situation?	☐	☐

Did you give any of the following:

	Yes	No
a) Personalised leaflet ·	☐	☐
b) *Coping with Cancer* ·	☐	☐
c) *Help Is there* ·	☐	☐
d) Information on specific cancer ·	☐	☐
e) Other (please specify)		

Please return to Gay Walker, Lynda Jackson Macmillan Centre for Cancer Support and Information

Appendix 5

Audit procedure

LYNDA JACKSON MACMILLAN CENTRE FOR CANCER SUPPORT AND INFORMATION

Communication Audit – Procedure for New Cancer Patients

When the clinic nurse becomes aware that a patient is about to be given a diagnosis of cancer for the first time, she will put the following documents into the notes

- audit form
- personalised leaflet – with sticker on the front
- *Help Is There*
- *Coping with Cancer*

Once the doctor has seen the patient, the nurse will complete the second side of the form and send it to Gay Walker at the Lynda Jackson MacMillan Centre.